CONSUMER GUIDE

CALCIUM COUNTER

Contributing Editors
Sara Silverman Rhodes, R.D.
Roger Field, Health and Science Editor/ NBC Radio Network

Cover Design
Terese Kolodziej

CONTENTS

INTRODUCTION

Once thought to be little more than a boring component of the human diet, calcium recently rocketed into public prominence as the darling food supplement of the 1980's. Lately, hardly a month passes without a feature on calcium surfacing in the women's magazines. Television news reports now often focus on the benefits of calcium. Even the stodgy, sometimes doubting medical profession is taking a new look at this ancient element. Like sodium in the 1970's, calcium has become the single most debated food supplement of the present decade. Antacid manufacturers boast that their products contain it. The dairy industry has stopped touting the protein content of its milks, creams, and cheeses to boast about their calcium content instead. Even a major soft-drink company is contemplating the addition of calcium in order to boost sales of a diet cola that has gone flat in the marketplace. In just two years, sales of calcium supplements have skyrocketed from $47 million to $125 million; sales are expected to reach $200 million next year.

Why all the hoopla? Behind the rush to gobble calcium are several surprising findings, all centering on this one inexpensive substance. The first spurt of interest came in April 1984, when a panel of experts assembled by the National Institutes of Health listed calcium (along with the female hormone estrogen) as the main way elderly people can prevent the devastating effects of developing brittle bones—a condition known as *osteoporosis*. With more Americans than ever before over the age of 65, this was important news indeed.

Since 1984, calcium deficiency has been tied to several other unrelated ailments. *Gum disease,* which affects 90 percent of the American population at some point in life, may be caused in part by too little calcium. Recent studies suggest a lack of sufficient calcium may also play a role in certain forms of *hypertension*—high blood pressure—an ailment affecting more than 60 million Americans. Thus, increasing calcium intake for some people might help them avoid heart attacks and strokes. The latest calcium connection suggests a possible role in preventing colorectal cancer—the second most prevalent cancer in this country. Little wonder that everybody's suddenly interested in calcium.

Why we all need calcium

The average person is walking around with approximately 2½ pounds of calcium. Some 99 percent of it is in the bones. They are strong and firm because they're made of a honeycomb structure largely formed of calcium along with another element, phosphorus, and protein fibers called *collagen.* But without the calcium, none of us could stand up or take a single step; our fragile skeletons would collapse under the weight of the rest of the body.

Although this may hardly seem possible, the remaining one percent of calcium in our bodies is even more important. Calcium plays a part in maintaining proper heart rhythm. It helps blood to clot when we're cut. It keeps us in motion by regulating muscle contractions. It also helps transmit nerve impulses. And it's the main ingredient in the dentin and enamel that make up our teeth.

As if all that weren't enough, calcium plays a role in the chemical activities of the basic cells that comprise our skin and organs. And it acts as a "glue" in binding cells together. Without that crucial one percent of calcium in your cells and bloodstream, your heart wouldn't beat, your muscles wouldn't move, and your brain wouldn't think.

What happens when you don't get enough calcium?

Because of calcium's crucial role in the cells and bloodstream, when you don't get enough calcium in your diet, your body attempts to maintain needed levels in your blood and cells by "borrowing" calcium from your calcium warehouse—your bones. One reason your mother urged you as a child to drink your milk every day was to build those strong bones. But even she may not have realized how crucial the calcium content of that milk would be in later life. People who don't store up enough calcium in their growing years, break bones with the slightest fall starting as early as their 50's, especially if dietary deficiencies have steadily robbed calcium from their skeletal systems for decades. Loss of supporting bone structure in the mouth has been known to erode away support for teeth, resulting in tooth loss. Preliminary studies suggest that chronic calcium deficiencies may more than double a genetically susceptible person's tendency to develop polyps and tumors of the colon. For about one-third of the 60 million Americans with high blood pressure, inadequate calcium intake may be responsible for some of their hypertension. In short, 42 percent of all Americans—a staggering total of 96 million of us—are taking in less than 70 percent of the modest recommended daily allowance of calcium each day. And many of us are paying for this calcium deficiency with our health and our lives.

How much calcium should we take?

How much calcium is ideal for you depends on how old you are, whether you are male or female, and—if female—whether you are past menopause, pregnant, or breast-feeding a child. In addition, expert opinion on how much dietary calcium is necessary keeps changing, generally inching higher as newer scientific studies and data come in.

The official estimate for calories and essential nutrients like calcium is revised every five years or so and published as a list of Recommended Dietary Allowances (RDAs). These come from the Food and Nutrition Board of the National Research Council, which, in turn, is part of the National Academy of Sciences—an agency of the federal government. The figures it contains are intended for groups of people, classified by sex and age, not for specific individuals. And, clearly, the figures represent the best advice available at the time they're issued (in RDA, the "R" stands for *Recommended,* not *Required.*) The most recent RDAs were issued in 1980. Although new RDAs were due to be released in 1985, they were postponed at least a year because of scientific disagreements over some of the figures.

The RDAs include a generous margin of safety, thus, they greatly exceed the minimum amount of nutrients needed to prevent scurvy, rickets, and other obvious disorders caused by nutritional deficiencies. Although they do allow for individual variations, the RDAs are basically set to meet the needs of healthy people. Nutritional needs are readily affected by certain illnesses and medications. All this considered, the RDAs are used as a nutritional yardstick—to measure adequate amounts of nutrients consumed by groups of people, including military troops, children served by school lunch programs, and senior citizens taking part in the National Nutrition Program for the

Elderly. The figures for all these groups are summarized into one number—generally the highest figure available—for use on food labels (where manufacturers simply do not have space to give several figures for each nutrient in a given product). The number cited on food labels is called the "U.S. RDA." For calcium, the U.S. RDA for adults is set at 1,000 milligrams a day. This is an amount of pure calcium equal to approximately one-tenth the weight of an ordinary penny. In fact, the RDAs for calcium range from 360 milligrams (for infants) to 1,600 milligrams a day (for pregnant and breast-feeding teenagers). But there is reason to believe that somewhat higher doses would be better.

Calcium: a readily available material

In its pure form, calcium is actually a silver-white, relatively soft metal. It is the fifth most abundant chemical element in the Earth's crust. But it isn't found in nature in its pure form; rather, it combines with other elements to form limestone, marble, dolomite, chalk, or pearl. You also find calcium in most plant and animal tissue. It is the fifth most abundant element in the human body as well. Our bones are tough and rigid because they are made of a honeycomb structure formed when calcium and phosphorus combine to create a hard mineral called *apatite*. Infant bones are relatively soft, because they have yet to take on much of their calcium. Gradually, through childhood and adolescence, they acquire more calcium phosphate until the age of 35, when the skeleton reaches its maximum weight, size, and toughness. During those 35 years the body's total content of calcium grows from one ounce in newborns to more than 2½ pounds in adults. During periods of rapid growth—in early adolescence—the growing child adds one full ounce of new calcium *every week*!

In our mid-thirties, the process is reversed and our bones start losing calcium. In a sense, our bones are the calcium warehouse—or storage facility—of the human body. Bone is a living material—at all ages it is simultaneously losing atoms of calcium and gaining other atoms of calcium. It is generally true that for the first 35 years of your life, calcium gains outpace calcium losses, and the net effect is to build bone. After age 35, the situation reverses for a net loss each year of calcium and bone. During this period, a healthy woman loses approximately one percent of the bone mass in her spine and pelvis each year. A male loses bone and calcium at about half that rate. Then loss of bone accelerates after age 50, especially in women, following menopause.

Clearly, the goal is to bank as much bone and calcium as you can before age 35, then hold losses after that to a minimum.

How to keep your calcium

Some people build big, solid bones easily, and lose bone very, very slowly. Others never develop anything more than a frail skeleton, and rapidly lose what little calcium they have. Clearly, the genes you get from your father and mother at conception play an important role in the development of ailments due to calcium deficiency. Hormonal and environmental factors also make a difference. Exercise—especially weight-bearing exercise such as walking, jogging, and running—is believed to help build bone in your formative years, and slow or stop bone loss after age 35. Conversely, resting in bed without moving day after day definitely accelerates bone loss.

The female hormone estrogen also plays a role. Contrary to early belief, having several children may actually protect a woman from too much bone loss. Pregnancy probably prevents fractures; it certainly doesn't cause them. Estrogen levels and the body's efficiency in handling calcium increase during pregnancy, thereby promoting bone formation. Still, women—because they generally possess smaller bones than men and because their hormone levels change substantially at menopause—are more likely than men to suffer debilitating bone thinning and the devastating effects of severe calcium loss.

The effects of calcium deficiency

By far, the best understood consequence of severe, chronic calcium deficiency is brittle bones—*osteoporosis*. One out of every four women over the age of 60 suffers from this disorder. Osteoporosis is a major cause of fractures of the hip, spine, ribs, and wrist.

At highest risk are white women who are small-boned, underweight, post-menopausal, and genetically prone to this disorder, especially those women who had their ovaries removed early in life. Men may also develop osteoporosis, although they are less prone to do so because of their denser bone structure.

Although the exact cause of osteoporosis is still unknown, these risk factors are clear: estrogen shortage (in women), inadequate calcium in the diet, smoking, and lack of physical activity. Regular, heavy use of products that can prevent the body from absorbing dietary calcium can also lead to osteoporosis. These include excess salt, caffeine, and nicotine. Certain medications can also block calcium absorption, including the antibiotic *tetracycline*, *corticosteroids*, a blood thinner called *heparin*, and a diuretic named *furosemide*. In addition, diabetes, alcoholism, and eating too much protein or fiber can reduce calcium absorption.

Osteoporosis is called "the silent epidemic" because it progresses gradually, and at first, painlessly. Moreover, calcium loss from the bones doesn't show up on X-rays until at least 25 percent is gone, at which time irreversible damage has already occurred. The first noticeable symptoms of this disorder are chronic backache and loss of height—sometimes as much as six or eight inches. Eventually, bones in the spine compress and fracture, leading to a curving of the upper back known as the "dowager's hump." In advanced stages, the bones become so brittle that they fracture under the slightest pressure of any sudden move.

In its most severe form, osteoporosis has been known to result in cracked ribs when the patient attempts to rise out of a chair. Sneezing has been shown to cause multiple fractures of the spine. And osteoporosis is a major cause of death for older women in the United States. The ailment afflicts an estimated 20 million Americans—mostly women over 45—and results in well over a million bone fractures a year. Of those women suffering a fracture of the hip, one out of every five—some 40,000 a year—dies of complications.

Treatment of osteoporosis consists of trying to stem further bone loss, often by prescribing calcium supplements with added vitamin D, and sometimes estrogen and fluoride. But excessive fluoride can be toxic. And estrogen therapy has been associated with increased risk of uterine cancer.

Bad gums and loss of teeth

Chronic calcium deficiency can also cause you to lose your teeth. Cavities used to be blamed exclusively on diets rich in sweets and poor teeth-cleaning habits, leading to the formation of gummy plaque. Bacteria present within the plaque generate acid that eats through tooth surfaces, thus causing cavities. But some researchers are beginning to include a newly recognized factor—insufficient calcium, causing soft teeth that are prone to decay.

The calcification of teeth actually begins while the fetus is still in the womb, at about the 14th week of pregnancy. Even the permanent teeth begin to calcify long before they can be seen—as early as the fourth month of life and continuing into the early twenties. Insufficient calcium intake during this entire period can result in poorly calcified teeth that are prone to cavities.

The high blood pressure connection

Sixty million Americans have high blood pressure, which greatly increases their risk of heart attack and stroke. Although scientists do not know the exact cause of this condition, risk factors include high salt (sodium) intake, being overweight, heredity, smoking cigarettes, and physical inactivity. And the beginnings of a connection are being made to low calcium consumption. In at least one study, people with high blood pressure were found to consume significantly less calcium than those with normal blood pressure.

Another calcium connection to high blood pressure comes from studies of hypertension and water hardness. Drinking water is considered hard if it has high levels of two minerals: calcium and magnesium. Years ago, scientists working in Britain discovered a relationship between heart disease death rates and water hardness. In general, the lower the death rate, the harder the water.

The next step was to investigate death rates from heart disease where water systems changed hardness levels over a period of years. The association between hard water and lower death rates was confirmed. Where water had become harder—that is, where it contained increasing concentrations of calcium and magnesium—death rates decreased. Where it got softer, death rates increased.

A recent study in Canada confirmed the relationship on this side of the Atlantic. Heart attack deaths were found to be at least 20 percent more frequent in a city with soft water than in one with hard water.

While more research is needed before the connection is proved, research clearly suggests that hard water may have a favorable effect on the heart.

The new connection: colorectal cancer

If beneficial effects of increased calcium on heart disease and a major bone ailment weren't enough, the most recent scientific revelation surrounding calcium centers on cancer—specifically cancer of the colon and rectum. Again calcium seems to have a beneficial effect. As reported in the *New England Journal of Medicine*, researchers Martin Lipkin, M.D. and Harold Newman, M.S. studied the tendency of certain people to grow cancer-prone colon cells.

Specifically, ten participants at high risk of developing colon cancer (because of family history) were given 1,250 milligrams of calcium supplement per day, in addition to approximately 700 milligrams of dietary calcium. It was found that the tendency to grow cancer-prone cells in these participants was significantly reduced. Scientists still don't know how the calcium influenced the growth of these cells. One possible explanation is that calcium may make the fatty acids and bile acids normally found in the bowel less irritating, but this is only a theory. Much more work needs to be done before researchers can conclusively state that calcium prevents cancer of the colon. And nobody is saying that calcium has any useful role in curing or treating colon cancers. But additional research may eventually confirm a possible role for calcium as one factor in reducing the risk of colorectal cancer in healthy people.

Helping your body use calcium efficiently

In addition to the possible hazard of forming kidney stones, eating too much calcium—especially supplements sold in pill form—can be a colossal waste of money. That's because your body eliminates excess calcium in its bodily waste. In fact, people vary enormously in their ability to absorb and use calcium, depending on age, sex, and heredity.

Men absorb calcium more efficiently than women, which probably helps explain why fewer men suffer from osteoporosis in later years. Absorption is much more efficient during childhood and adolescence than later in life. Up to 75 percent of the calcium children take in is absorbed by their bodies, whereas young and middle-aged adults absorb between 20 and 30 percent of their intake. The most dramatic decrease comes later: calcium absorption drops sharply for women after age 40; for men after age 60. For example, post-menopausal women may only absorb seven percent of the calcium they consume. This is believed to be due to declining levels of certain hormones—in particular, estrogen.

The variability of calcium absorption may well serve as a safety valve to prevent calcium overdose. When calcium is supplied abundantly for many years, the body's efficiency in absorbing that calcium declines; where calcium intake is low for prolonged periods, the body compensates by absorbing it more efficiently.

Maintaining steady intake is important. When a well-nourished American moves to a country where there is no milk, for example, he may suffer from calcium deficiency. By contrast, natives living in that same country, who are long accustomed to the lack of dairy products, may have strong bones and be perfectly healthy.

Then, too, what we eat along with the calcium may well affect how much of it is absorbed. Vitamin D helps our bodies absorb calcium more than any other nutrient that plays a role in calcium absorption. We get most of the vitamin D in our diet from fortified milk and milk products, and from fish liver oils. Your body also produces some of its own vitamin D when your skin absorbs sunlight.

If you are deficient in vitamin D, calcium encounters difficulty passing through the intestinal wall, into your bloodstream, and on to your muscles, bones, and teeth. That's why children who don't get enough vitamin D get rickets—an ailment characterized by weakened bones and bowed legs. Similarly, adults who don't get enough vitamin D invite a condition known as *osteomalacia*—in which their calcium-deprived bones become brittle and fracture easily.

Vitamin D also regulates your body's ability to obtain calcium from its storage in bones. It aids the building of strong teeth. And it helps your body hold on to the calcium it needs by preventing calcium excretion. However, it is generally not prudent to take supplements of vitamin D because your body does make this nutrient, and large doses can be toxic.

Lactose—the main carbohydrate in milk—is another nutrient that speeds and aids the body's absorption of calcium. Indeed, milk is the best source of lactose, especially skim milk and powdered milk. Other dairy products also contain lactose, but generally in lower concentrations. For example, the lactose levels in yogurt are low, because the bacteria that make yogurt digest some of the lactose. Production also causes loss of lactose in the making of cheese: the whey—a byproduct of the cheese-making process—carries off much of the lactose when it is separated from the curd.

Phosphorus also helps the body absorb calcium, in part because you need both elements to build bone. Fortunately, both calcium and phosphorus are found together in some dairy products. Nutritionists differ on what ratio of calcium to phosphorus is ideal, but most agree that a ratio somewhat higher in calcium is preferred—say, about 2:1 of calcium to phosphorus. On the other hand, animal studies suggest that too much phosphorus in the diet can lead to a loss of calcium, although this effect has not yet been seen in people. Still, for this reason, some authorities fear that diets high in phosphorus—from consuming lots of meat and soft drinks—might interfere with calcium absorption. Other experts remain unconvinced that excessive phosphorus has a significant effect on calcium uptake.

Other nutritional components affect calcium absorption, as do certain living habits. Some experts believe that vitamin C and two amino acids—*lysine* and *arginine*—increase calcium uptake. Exposure to sunlight and regular physical exercise are known to improve it.

On the other hand, a lack of exercise, excessive consumption of certain nutrients, and even some medications can accelerate a *loss* of calcium, as well as interfere with calcium absorption.

Excessive alcohol consumption is especially detrimental. For this reason, osteoporosis occurs earlier in alcoholics than those who drink in moderation. Of course, alcoholics often have poor eating habits, due in part to depressed appetites, so intake of dietary calcium is often low as well. In addition, alcohol itself inhibits the absorption of calcium and may be toxic to bone formation.

Caffeine—present in most coffees, teas, and colas—can also interfere with calcium uptake. While drinking a cup of tea or coffee, or a glass of cola every day is of no concern, heavy and steady consumption of caffeinated beverages could prevent your body from putting to use the calcium you obtain from your diet.

Even a diet high in protein may cause urinary elimination of calcium. One possible explanation for some of the osteoporosis so widespread in this country is that Americans eat a diet rich in protein. Our eating habits may contribute to calcium loss. Most nutritionists agree that protein intake in healthy people should not exceed 15 percent of total calories. Under normal circumstances, there is no benefit to protein ingestion beyond this amount: the excess is burned for energy or stored as fat.

Excessive fat in the diet can also interfere with calcium uptake, by causing the formation of insoluble calcium compounds that are excreted. For many reasons, not just this one, it's important to remember that your diet should contain no more than 30 percent fat. High fat consumption is increasingly being tied to heart disease, stroke, and possibly colon cancer.

To some degree, the current vogue of emphasizing fiber in the diet may affect the calcium available to your body and bones. *Oxalic acid*—a component of beet greens, Swiss chard, and spinach—binds to calcium, reducing its ability to be absorbed. Be aware that these vegetables appear in nutrition charts to be high in calcium, but not all the calcium present in these sources is necessarily available to your body. Precisely the same problem crops up with bran and whole-grain cereals. These contain a food component called *phytic acid* that binds calcium, making it unavailable for use. This is not to say that dietary fiber should be avoided; it certainly has an important place in a healthy diet. There's no reason to forever banish bananas, bran muffins, or peanuts from your pantry. On the other hand, excessive amounts of bran and whole grains—such as those used in macrobiotic diets—would best be avoided.

Some medications can affect the way your body handles calcium. Certainly, thyroid drugs, diuretics (water pills), and laxatives can hinder calcium absorption. The commonly prescribed antibiotic *tetracycline,* antacids containing aluminium, and a drug to treat tuberculosis called *isoniazid* can all lead to loss of bone with regular use.

In addition, some medical conditions tend to bring on bone loss, regardless of what medications are used to treat them. Prolonged immobilization, paralysis, diabetes, celiac disease (an intestinal disorder characterized by an intolerance of dietary gluten), and chronic kidney failure can all decrease calcium absorption.

Whether you're healthy or not, there are ways to improve calcium absorption. Here are some tips you may wish to consider:

• Consume dairy products, especially those high in calcium and low in butterfat (cholesterol) such as skim milk and powdered milk. Milk contains lactose and is fortified with vitamin D, both of which aid calcium absorption and have excellent calcium-to-phosphorous ratios. Other dairy products that could be beneficial include ice milk, sherbet, cottage cheese, and buttermilk.

• Try to select low-fat dairy products where you can. If you wish to eat cheese, for example, choose ricotta cheese, Jarlsberg cheese, mozzarella made with skim milk, and low-fat cottage cheese.

• Endeavor to eat dairy products together with foods rich in vitamin C, such as strawberries with milk or an orange with milk.

• Limit the fat in your diet. You can do this by selecting lean cuts of meat, broiling or steaming foods rather than frying them, removing the skin of chicken or turkey before cooking. Also, try broiling or baking lean fish, and substituting bread or matzos for croissants or buttery buns.

• Limit your intake of beverages that are high in caffeine, including coffee, tea, and cola.

• Keep moving. Walking, jogging, and running really do strengthen bones.

• Limit your consumption of alcohol. Virtually every nutrient—including calcium—is adversely affected by excessive alcohol. At the most, drink two or three one-ounce cocktails a day, or the same number of beers or glasses of wine.

• If possible, breast-feed your baby. Obviously, this doesn't apply if you're a man. Babies benefit from breast-feeding—despite the fact that breast milk is slightly lower in calcium than cow's milk (because breast milk is rich in lactose and vitamin C). The calcium that the baby gets is better absorbed.

• Cut out—or at least cut down—big steak dinners washed down with soda pop. Such meals are as outdated as the hula hoop. Keep your protein and phosphorus intake under tight control.

Should you use a calcium supplement?

Many people are starting to make up for any shortage of calcium in their diet by taking supplemental calcium in the form of tablets, capsules, or special liquids. But which type is best for you? And how much should you be taking? To help determine how much calcium supplement you need, use the handy tables in this book to estimate how much calcium you consume in your diet. The best way to do that is to keep a three-day food record that includes one weekend day. Don't forget to add in the milk or cream you add to your coffee, tea, or cereal. To arrive at your daily intake, simply add up all the calcium you take in during the three days you're keeping your log, then divide by three. It's that simple!

Next, refer to Table 1—Recommended Dietary Allowances (RDAs)—and see how much calcium experts presently think you should be getting. Then compare your actual average with what you should be taking in. Are you getting enough calcium? If not, you can change your diet to include more calcium-rich food. And you can make up any remaining difference by taking calcium supplements.

As you might suspect, it's generally better to get your calcium from food rather than supplements (pills). For one thing, your body absorbs calcium more readily from food than from supplements. Also, the pills may cause some unpleasant side effects. Supplements containing calcium carbonate—the most common supplement ingredient—may cause constipation, or worse yet, kidney stones if taken to excess by susceptible individuals. Pills containing calcium chloride may irritate the stomach. In addition, calcium supplements often are chalky, and some are unpleasant tasting or hard to swallow. They also can be bulky, because calcium must be combined with another ingredient (such as carbonate, chloride, citronate, or gluconate) to be absorbed. This, combined with an inert binder to hold the tablet together, often yields a pretty big pill that doesn't have all that much calcium. So you may have to take several tablets to get your daily quota. And having to remember to take that many tablets, often at various times during the day, is a drawback. Then again, pills containing multiple vitamins and minerals have very little calcium, so trying to shore up your calcium intake with those pills could result in toxic overdoses of vitamins.

But the supplements do have a place when used intelligently. People who do not tolerate lactose, and therefore cannot drink milk, may well profit from supplements, as would those who find most foods high in calcium unappetizing. And many people find the supplements a handy way to make up for modest differences in what they can reasonably get from foods each day, and what they ought to be taking in.

A word of warning: calcium supplements are not to be taken by people susceptible to formation of kidney stones, certainly not without first consulting a physician. And do not give calcium supplements to children unless their doctor specifies that you do so. Those taking medications should also check with their doctor before taking calcium supplements.

What supplements are available?

There are so many different forms of calcium supplements on the market today that choosing one may seem like a confusing task. Your choices include calcium carbonate, gluconate, citrate, lactate, and dicalcium phosphate, among others. The pure calcium is always combined with another salt or compound. Figure 1 shows you the relative amounts of calcium contained in various supplement formulas. Use the chart to figure out how much calcium you'll be getting. For example, since calcium carbonate is just 40 percent calcium (and 60 percent carbonate), a 500 milligram tablet actually contains just 200 milligrams of calcium. Reckon by the 200 milligrams of pure calcium when figuring how much supplement you will need. For example, if your RDA for calcium is 1,200 milligrams and your log indicates that you're getting 800 milligrams a day, you'll need 400 milligrams more of calcium, or a total of two pills, containing 500 milligrams of calcium carbonate each, because each tablet actually contains 200 milligrams of pure calcium.

The various forms of calcium are assimilated by the body about equally well, according to a report in the April, 1985 *Tufts University Diet and Nutrition Letter* ("Picking the right calcium supplement"). Supplements are available as liquids, powders, tablets, and capsules. A survey by Tufts University compared seven supplements for cost, proportion of calcium, and safety. By these standards, *calcium carbonate* was rated best. It's available in some antacids, in particular, Tums. It also comes as a synthetic product, but is usually made from crushed oyster shells. All these forms contain about 40 percent calcium. Tufts reports that calcium carbonate sold as antacids is virtually identical to that sold as calcium supplements. According to the report, an antacid like Tums that is taken in doses recommended on its package label should not upset the body's acid-base balance. However, the Tufts researchers found that 8 to 16 Tums taken at the same time actually stimulates, rather than suppresses, stomach acid secretion. Therefore, doses of calcium carbonate should be spread out through the day, rather than all at once. Also keep in mind that not all antacids contain calcium carbonate: for example, Rolaids, DiGel, Maalox, Mylanta, and Gelusil contain aluminum, not calcium. You may wish to avoid calcium supplements containing bone meal or dolomite because they may contain lead or mercury, both of which are toxic.

In any case, megadoses of calcium supplements are not recommended. According to researchers reporting in the *American Journal of Clinical Nutrition*, healthy people should not take more than 2,500 milligrams of calcium per day.

Finding calcium in our land of milk and molasses

As children, we were just told to drink our milk. Today, children are advised to eat their tofu and yogurt as well to meet their calcium needs. Understanding how to get adequate calcium and a well-balanced diet in this world of fast foods, convenience foods, and foreign foods has become a much more complicated and challenging task.

Calcium is found in all four of the major food groups (see Figure 2). Dairy products are the richest source of this mineral. Milk, cheese, yogurt, ice milk, and some other dairy foods are good choices. They contain high levels of calcium, as well as lactose and vitamin D that help the calcium get absorbed. Butter and cream, however, are poor sources of calcium, since it doesn't dissolve in fat. To obtain the amount of calcium in one cup of milk, you would have to consume 10 eggs, 5 pounds of roast beef, 22 doughnuts, 448 french fried potatoes, 30 apples, 97 hot dogs, 3 pounds of butter, 2 quarts of rosé wine, or 6 quarts of beer. Clearly, none of these mega-calorie options is the answer to solving a calcium deficiency.

Some alternative sources of protein and calcium that do make sense include salmon and canned sardines (including the bones). In fact, the soft, edible bones contain most of the calcium in these foods. Shellfish also contain quite a bit of calcium, as does some tofu because it's processed with calcium sulfate.

Green, leafy vegetables are also good sources of calcium. Kale, turnip greens, mustard greens, bok choy, and dandelion greens are good choices in this category. However, keep in mind that their calcium is not completely absorbed because these vegetables also contain *oxalic acid,* which inhibits calcium uptake by the body. Because they generally contain negligible amounts of calcium, fruits would be a poor choice. But there are exceptions. Oranges, for example, each contain 52 milligrams of the mineral.

Reportedly, calcium levels of breads and cereals depend on the grain they are made from, the processing methods used, and the degree of enrichment of ingredients. For example, whole wheat flour contains more than twice the amount of calcium found in white flour. In general, breads and cereals are relatively low in calcium.

Among the starchy foods there are surprises. Blackstrap molasses is loaded with calcium; just two tablespoons contain about the same amount of calcium you would find in a cup of milk.

Tips to boost the calcium you get from food

It's not all that difficult. By shopping right and eating right you *can* increase the amount of calcium-rich food in your diet. Here are some suggestions:

- Use milk—especially skim or powdered milk—instead of water when you prepare soups.
- Instead of coffee or tea, try cocoa.
- Prepare casseroles and sauces with skim or powdered milk.
- Enjoy low-fat cheese instead of candy or nuts as a snack. Make macaroni and cheese, or cheese sandwiches, with cheeses that are relatively low in fat and reasonably high in calcium. But remember: the cholesterol content of cheese can be a problem, especially if you are prone to atherosclerosis or have a high blood cholesterol count.
- Have ice cream, custard, or pudding for dessert, or better yet, ice milk or frozen yogurt. Generally, the cheaper brands of ice cream have less cream and therefore less butterfat, and are healthier than the premium brands.
- For salads, use spinach, collard greens, and other dark green, leafy vegetables instead of head lettuce.

• Place fresh strawberries or peaches in your blender and combine with yogurt to make interesting high calcium desserts. Or mix applesauce with yogurt and cinnamon. Because you can control the amount of sugar added to these yogurt-based desserts, you can hold down the calories. It's not difficult to prepare them with fewer calories than those commercial yogurt products containing sugar-laden fruit preserves.

• Make a milkshake, or frappe (as it's called in some parts of the country), by blending fruit with milk, ice cream, or ice milk. Or mix yogurt, a little blackstrap molasses, a piece of banana, and some chopped ice in a blender; voila, a refreshing, high-calcium shake!

Since some of these suggestions hinge on milk or other dairy products that contain lactose, here are some tips for those of you suffering from a lactose intolerance—a disorder characterized by the deficiency of an enzyme, lactase, that normally breaks down lactose (milk sugar) so it can be absorbed by the body.

There are lactose-free milk products and soy milk, either of which can be used in place of cow's milk. In addition, there are special tablets and drops—sold under the brand name *Lact-Aid*—that can be added to ordinary milk to help digest the lactose. Check with your doctor to see if you can safely try it. Some people with lactose intolerance can drink unaltered, regular milk in small amounts. Others with this disorder may have yogurt; hard cheese; dark green, leafy vegetables; tofu (bean curd); and canned sardines or salmon.

Use the charts to find the right calcium-rich foods for you

Vegetarians who drink milk and eat dairy products—so-called lacto-vegetarians—can easily meet their calcium needs. Strict vegans (vegetarians who don't eat any dairy foods, eggs, meat, fish, or chicken) are advised by the American Dietetic Association to drink fortified soy milk, and eat dark green, leafy vegetables as well as nuts—especially filberts and almonds. Fortified soy milk can usually be found in the baby food section of your grocery store. Vegans might wish to consult with a registered dietitian to select appropriate foods that are rich in calcium.

People who are dieting to lose weight can readily meet their calcium needs by selecting skim or low-fat dairy products like low-fat cottage cheese. The dietary key to weight control is to limit fats, sugar, and alcohol, and select fresh vegetables, fruits, fish, poultry (without the skin), and lean cuts of meat. And, of course, eat modest portions.

Guidelines for each age group

Youngsters up to the age of 10 should try to include at least three servings of calcium-rich food in their diet each day. Preteens and teenagers need four servings. If you're between the ages of 19 and 40, you also need four servings. The recommendation for older adults, especially post-menopausal women, is five servings of high-calcium foods. Pregnant and breast-feeding women also need five servings a day.

It's not all that hard to get adequate calcium just from food. Since one cup of milk contains 300 milligrams of calcium, you can obtain 900 a day just by drinking three cups—say, one with each meal. By adding an additional ½ cup of yogurt or one tablespoon of blackstrap molasses, you'll easily attain the ideal 1,000 milligram level for most adults. (See Table 2, Calcium Exchanges, for milk substitutes that are approximately equivalent in calcium content to milk.) If you dislike milk, you can still attain the 1,000 milligram figure by eating two ounces of Swiss cheese, one cup of collard greens, and one cup of ice milk. Creative use of this guide allows numerous possibilities for adding variety to your diet, while meeting your calcium needs.

Above all, you should enjoy eating calcium-rich foods. Don't view them as something you *have* to eat in order to ward off the scourge of disease. Eating nutritiously should be a pleasurable experience. Furthermore, it need not be especially expensive. In fact, for people watching their pennies, money expended on calcium supplement pills (some of which are quite expensive) can certainly be better invested in foods that contain calcium and lots of other nutrients. Generally, food provides calcium that is more easily assimilated and stored. And food looks better on the dining room table than a handful of pills!

How to use the calcium counter

Here are some tips that will help you use the calcium listing that follows. Start by looking up your Recommended Dietary Allowance for intake of calcium in Table 1. Experts believe that a reasonable maximum for calcium consumption under nor-

TABLE 1

Recommended Dietary Allowances (RDAs) for Calcium

CHILDREN AND ADULTS:

Age	*Milligrams/Day*
0-0.5 yr	360
0.5-1.0 yr	540
1-10 yr	800
10-18 yr	1,200
19+ yr	800
Post-menopausal women	1,500 (proposed)
PREGNANT AND BREAST-FEEDING WOMEN:	
10-18 yr	1,600
19+ yr	1,200

TABLE 2

CALCIUM EXCHANGES

The following foods contain 300 milligrams of calcium:

1 cup of milk or buttermilk
1½ oz of cheddar cheese
1 oz of Swiss cheese
1½ oz of American cheese
2½ cups of cottage cheese
1¾ cups of ice milk or ice cream
½ cup of ricotta cheese, part-skim
1 cup of yogurt
20 medium oysters
4 oz of canned salmon with bones
2¼ oz of sardines with bones
8 oz of tofu processed with calcium
1 cup of collard greens
2 tbsp of blackstrap molasses

mal circumstances for a healthy adult is 2,500 milligrams a day. More than that could be unhealthy.

Next, take a good look at Table 2, which shows calcium exchanges. It lists 14 foods—all reasonably high in calcium—and the size of a portion that yields 300 milligrams of calcium.

Figure 1
Calcium Content of Some Common Calcium Supplements

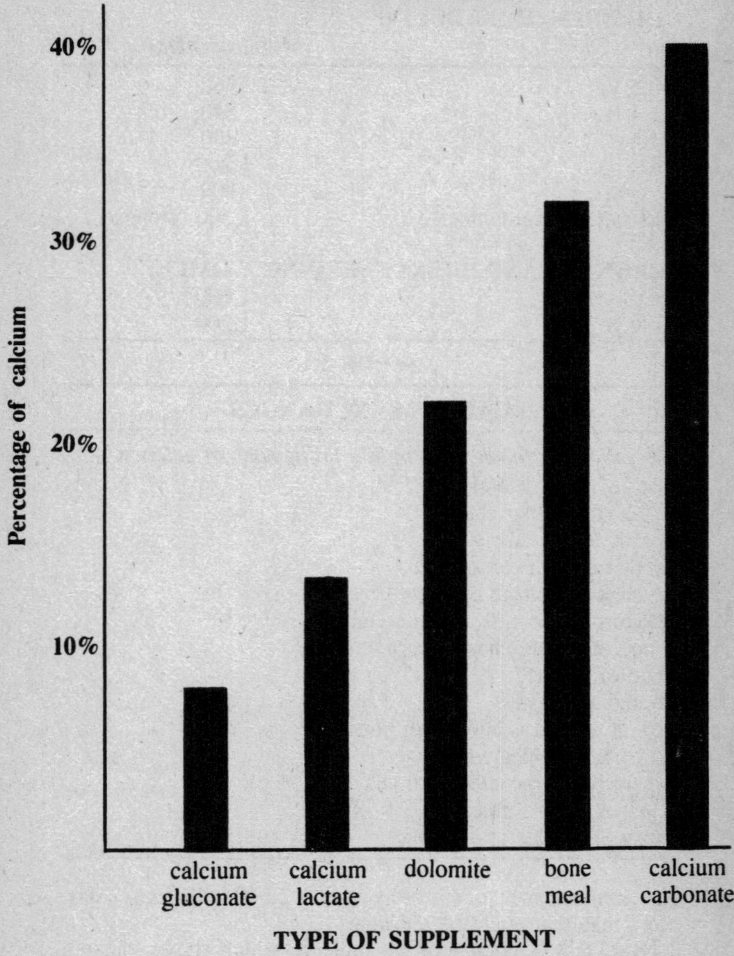

You might wish to jot down your favorites from this list on a slip of paper and take it to the supermarket the next time you shop. That way, you can make sure you have some high calcium foods at home that you can use in planning meals.

You are now ready to use the calcium counter. Please observe that calcium content varies by style of preparation. The figures for *cabbage*, for instance, varies from 18 to 37 milligrams for one-half cup depending on whether the cabbage is shredded, raw, red, Chinese, or cooked. And different brands of the same dish may have very different levels of calcium. For example, Van Camp's brand of spanish rice has 35 milligrams per cup; Lipton's has almost none. Where the listing includes the word "prepared," that means the estimate for calcium content is based on how the food is prepared when you follow directions on the label. Obviously, food that requires milk as an added ingredient is likely to have a greater calcium content than a dish that's made with water.

When an asterisk (*) appears in the calcium counter, it means that the particular food item contains less than two percent of the U.S. RDA (or 20 milligrams of calcium).

By now, you should have some idea of whether or not you're likely to need calcium supplements to meet your proper Recommended Dietary Allowance of calcium. Figure 1 helps you determine how much pure calcium there is in various compounds containing the mineral. For example, at 40 percent, a 500 milligram tablet of *calcium carbonate* actually contains just 200 milligrams of calcium; a 500 milligram pill of *calcium gluconate*, however, contains less than 50 milligrams of pure calcium. In shopping for calcium supplements, keep in mind that a roll of Tums contains 12 small disks that sell for about four to five cents each. And each disk has 500 milligrams of calcium carbonate that yields 200 milligrams of pure calcium. Compare any supplement to that for cost and calcium quantity—as a way to keep your supplement purchase effective and economical.

Now go to it; look up your RDA, use the calcium exchange chart when shopping and planning, check out the various brands of your favorite dishes for calcium content, decide whether or not to purchase calcium supplements, and good luck. May you and your family enjoy your calcium-balanced meals for years to come, and never break a bone!

DAIRY AND EGG PRODUCTS

Food	*Portion*	*Calcium (mg)*
CHEESE		
American Cheese Food	1 oz.	141
American Cheese Food, grated (Kraft)	1 oz	150
American Cheese Food, Process slices (Borden)	1 oz	150
American Cheese, Process slices (Borden)	1 oz	200
American Cheese Spread	1 oz	159
American Flavored Pasteurized Process Cheese Product Singles (Light n' Lively)	1 oz	200
American, Hot Pepper, Process (Sargento)	1 oz.	174
American (Land O'Lakes)	1 oz	150
American Pasteurized Process	1 oz.	174
American Pasteurized Process Cheese Food	1 oz	163
American Pasteurized Process Cheese Spread, Easy Cheese (Nabisco)	1 oz	100

Food	*Portion*	*Calcium (mg)*
Cheese, *continued*		
American Pasteurized Process Sharp Loaf (Kraft)	1 oz	200
American Pasteurized Process Sharp, slices (Kraft)	1 oz	150
American Pasteurized Process, slices (Deluxe)	1 oz	150
American Pasteurized Process, loaf (Deluxe)	1 oz	200
American Process Cheese Product, 8% milkfat slices, Lite-line (Borden)	1 oz	200
American Process Cheese Product, Reduced Sodium slices, Lite-line, (Borden)	1 oz	200
American Process Cheese Product, Sodium Lite slices, Lite-line (Borden)	1 oz	200
American Sharp Spread Pasteurized Process Cracker Snacks (Sargento)	1 oz.	174
American Singles Pasteurized Process Cheese Food (Kraft)	1 oz	150
American with Pimento Pasteurized Process Crackers Snacks (Sargento)	1 oz.	174
American/Swiss (Land O'Lakes)	1 oz	200
Blue	1 oz	150

Food	*Portion*	*Calcium (mg)*
Cheese, *continued*		
Blue (Kraft)	1 oz	150
Blue (Sargento)	1 oz	150
Brick	1 oz.	191
Brick (Kraft)	1 oz	200
Brick (Land O'Lakes)	1 oz	200
Brick (Sargento)	1 oz.	191
Brick Spread Pasteurized Process Cracker Snacks (Sargento)	1 oz	149
Brie	1 oz	52
Brie (Sargento)	1 oz	52
Burger (Sargento)	1 oz.	174
Camembert	1 oz.	110
Camembert, domestic, in 4 oz package, 3 wedges per package	1 wedge	40
Camembert (Sargento)	1 oz.	110
Caraway	1 oz.	191
Caraway (Kraft)	1 oz	150
Cheddar	1 oz	204
Cheddar Cheese Nuggets, Breaded (Banquet)	3 oz	328
Cheddar Cold Pack Cheese Food, Port Wine (Cracker Barrel)	1 oz	150
Cheddar Cold Pack Cheese Food, Sharp (Cracker Barrel)	1 oz	150
Cheddar Flavored Sharp Process Cheese Product Singles (Light n' Lively)	1 oz	200
Cheddar, Imitation (Sargento)	1 oz	200
Cheddar (Kraft)	1 oz	200
Cheddar (Land O'Lakes)	1 oz	200

Food	*Portion*	*Calcium (mg)*
Cheese, *continued*		
Cheddar, Pasteurized Process Cheese Spread, Easy Cheese (Nabisco)	1 oz	100
Cheddar, Queso de Papa (Sargento)	1 oz	204
Cheddar (Sargento)	1 oz	204
Cheddar, Sharp, New York (Sargento)	1 oz	204
Cheddar, Sharp, Nut Log (Sargento)	1 oz.	175
Cheddar, Sharp, Pasteurized Process Cheese Spread, Easy Cheese (Nabisco)	1 oz	100
Cheddar, Sharp, Process Cheese Product, 8% milkfat, slice, Lite-line (Borden)	1 oz	200
Cheddar'n Chive, Pasteurized Process Cheese Spread, Easy Cheese (Nabisco)	1 oz	100
Cheese Food, Pasteurized Process (Smokelle)	1 oz	200
Cheese Food, Pasteurized Process with Bacon (Kraft)	1 oz	150
Cheese Spread, American, Pasteurized Process (Kraft)	1 oz	150
Cheese Spread, Pasteurized Process (Cheez Whiz)	1 oz	150
Cheese Spread, Pasteurized Process, Mexican, hot (Velveeta)	1 oz	150

Food	*Portion*	*Calcium (mg)*
Cheese, *continued*		
Cheese Spread, Pimento, Pasteurized Process (Velveeta)	1 oz	150
Cheese Spread, Pineapple (Kraft)	1 oz	40
Cheese Spread, Relish (Kraft)	1 oz	20
Cheese Spread, Sharp, Pasteurized Process (Kraft)	1 oz	150
Cheese Spread, Sharp, Pasteurized Process (Squeez-A-Snak)	1 oz	150
Cheese Spread with Bacon, Pasteurized Process (Kraft)	1 oz	150
Cheese Spread with Bacon, Pasteurized Process (Squeez-A-Snak)	1 oz	150
Cheese Spread with Garlic, Pasteurized Process (Kraft)	1 oz	150
Cheese Spread with Jalapeno Peppers, Pasteurized Process (Cheez Whiz)	1 oz	150
Cheese Spread with Pimento, Pasteurized Process (Squeez-A-Snak)	1 oz	150
Cheez'n Crackers (Handi-Snaks)	1 package	100
Cheshire	1 oz	182
Co-Jack (Sargento)	1 oz	203
Colby	1 oz	194
Colby (Kraft)	1 oz	200

Food	Portion	Calcium (mg)
Cheese, *continued*		
Colby (Land O'Lakes)	1 oz	200
Colby Process Cheese Product, 8% milkfat, slices, Lite-line (Borden)	1 oz	200
Colby (Sargento)	1 oz	194
Cottage Cheese, 2% (Land O'Lakes)	4 oz	80
Cottage Cheese, 4% milkfat minimum (Borden)	1/2 cup	60
Cottage Cheese, creamed	4 oz	68
Cottage Cheese, dry curd	4 oz	36
Cottage Cheese (Land O'Lakes)	4 oz	60
Cottage Cheese, lowfat, 1% fat	4 oz	69
Cottage Cheese, lowfat, 2% fat	4 oz	77
Cottage Cheese, lowfat, Lite-line (Borden)	1/2 cup	60
Cream Cheese	1 oz	23
Cream Cheese (Philadelphia)	1 oz	20
Cream Cheese, soft (Philadelphia)	1 oz	20
Cream Cheese, whipped (Philadelphia)	1 oz	20
Cream Cheese with Apples and Cinnamon, soft (Philadelphia)	1 oz	20
Cream Cheese with Bacon and Horseradish, whipped (Philadelphia)	1 oz	20

Food	Portion	Calcium (mg)
Cheese, *continued*		
Cream Cheese with Blue Cheese, whipped (Philadelphia)	1 oz	60
Cream Cheese with Chives and Onion, soft (Philadelphia)	1 oz	20
Cream Cheese with Chives (Philadelphia)	1 oz	20
Cream Cheese with Chives, whipped (Philadelphia)	1 oz	20
Cream Cheese with Onions, whipped (Philadelphia)	1 oz	40
Cream Cheese with Peaches, soft (Philadelphia)	1 oz	20
Cream Cheese with Pimentos (Philadelphia)	1 oz	20
Cream Cheese with Pimentos, whipped (Philadelphia)	1 oz	40
Cream Cheese with Pineapple, soft (Philadelphia)	1 oz	20
Cream Cheese with Smoked Salmon, whipped (Philadelphia)	1 oz	20
Cream Cheese with Strawberries, soft (Philadelphia)	1 oz	20
Edam	1 oz	207
Edam (Kraft)	1 oz	150
Edam (Land O'Lakes)	1 oz	200
Edam (Sargento)	1 oz	207
Farmer's (Sargento)	1 oz	219
Feta	1 oz	140

Food	*Portion*	*Calcium (mg)*
Cheese, *continued*		
Feta (Sargento)	1 oz	140
Fontina	1 oz	156
Fontina (Sargento)	1 oz	156
Gargonzola (Sargento)	1 oz	150
Gjetost (Sargento)	1 oz.	113
Golden Velvet cheese spread (Land O'Lakes)	1 oz	150
Gouda	1 oz	198
Gouda (Kraft)	1 oz	150
Gouda (Land O'Lakes)	1 oz	200
Gouda (Sargento)	1 oz	198
Gruyere	1 oz	287
Gruyere (Sargento)	1 oz	287
Havarti (Sargento)	1 oz	228
Italian Blend, grated (Kraft)	1 oz	400
Italian Grated Blend of Swiss,Provolone,and Romano (Sargento)	1 oz	277
Jalapeno Cheese Food (Land O'Lakes)	1 oz	150
Jalapeno Singles Pasteurized Process Cheese Food (Kraft)	1 oz	150
Jarlsberg (Sargento)	1 oz	200
LaChedda Cheese Food (Land O'Lakes)	1 oz	150
Limburger	1 oz.	141
Limburger (Sargento)	1 oz.	141
Monterey	1 oz	212
Monterey Jack (Kraft)	1 oz	200
Monterey Jack (Land O'Lakes)	1 oz	200

Food	Portion	Calcium (mg)
Cheese, *continued*		
Monterey Jack Process Cheese Product, 8% milkfat, slices, Lite-line (Borden)	1 oz	200
Monterey Jack (Sargento)	1 oz	212
Monterey Jack Singles Pasteurized Process Cheese Food (Kraft)	1 oz	150
Monterey Jack with Jalapeno Peppers (Kraft)	1 oz	150
Mozzarella	1 oz	147
Mozzarella Cheese Nuggets, Breaded (Banquet)	3 oz	355
Mozzarella, Imitation (Sargento)	1 oz	250
Mozzarella, Low-Moisture, part skim (Land O'Lakes)	1 oz	200
Mozzarella, Low-Moisture (Casino)	1 oz	150
Mozzarella, Low-Moisture, part skim (Kraft)	1 oz	200
Mozzarella, Low-Moisture, part skim (Sargento)	1 oz	207
Mozzarella, Low-Moisture, whole milk (Sargento)	1 oz	163
Mozzarella, part skim	1 oz	183
Mozzarella, Pizza, Low-Moisture, part skim (Sargento)	1 oz	207
Mozzarella, String (Sargento)	1 oz	207

Food	Portion	Calcium (mg)
Cheese, *continued*		
Mozzarella, String, with Jalapeno Peppers, Low-Moisture, part skim (Kraft)	1 oz	200
Mozzarella, with Pizza Spices, Provolone, Romano, and Parmesan (Sargento)	1 oz	200
Muenster	1 oz	203
Muenster (Kraft)	1 oz	200
Muenster (Land O'Lakes)	1 oz	200
Muenster Process Cheese Product, 8% milkfat, slices, Lite-line (Borden)	1 oz	200
Muenster, Queso Blanco (Sargento)	1 oz	203
Muenster, Red Rind	1 oz	203
Nacho, Pasteurized Process Cheese Spread, Easy Cheese (Nabisco)	1 oz	100
Neufchatel	1 oz	21
Neufchatel (Kraft)	1 oz	20
Onion cheese food (Land O'Lakes)	1 oz	200
Parmesan and Romano blend (Sargento)	1 oz.	319
Parmesan, grated	1 tbsp.	69
Parmesan, grated (Kraft)	1 oz	400
Parmesan, hard	1 oz	336
Parmesan, Imitation (Sargento)	1 oz	30
Parmesan, Natural (Kraft)	1 oz	300
Parmesan (Sargento)	1 oz	336

Food	Portion	Calcium (mg)
Cheese, *continued*		
Pasteurized Process Cheese Food, Singles (Kraft)	1 oz	150
Pasteurized Process Cheese Food with Garlic (Kraft)	1 oz	200
Pepperoni Cheese Food (Land O'Lakes)	1 oz	150
Pimento, Pasteurized Process	1 oz.	174
Pimento, Pasteurized Process slices (Kraft)	1 oz	150
Pimento, Singles, Pasteurized Process Cheese Food (Kraft)	1 oz	150
Port du Salut	1 oz	184
Port Wine, Nut Log (Sargento)	1 oz	169
Pot (Sargento)	1 oz	77
Provolone	1 oz.	214
Provolone (Land O'Lakes)	1 oz	200
Provolone (Sargento)	1 oz.	214
Ricotta, made with part skim milk	½ cup	337
Ricotta, made with whole milk	½ cup	257
Ricotta, part skim (Sargento)	1 oz	51
Ricotta, whole milk and whey (Sargento)	1 oz	60
Ricotta, whole milk (Sargento)	1 oz	83
Romano	1 oz	302
Romano, grated (Kraft)	1 oz	350
Romano, Natural (Casino)	1 oz	250

Food	*Portion*	*Calcium (mg)*
Cheese, *continued*		
Romano, Pecorino (Sargento)	1 oz	302
Romano (Sargento)	1 oz	302
Roquefort	1 oz	188
Salami cheese food (Land O'Lakes)	1 oz	150
Scamorze, Low-Moisture, part skim (Kraft)	1 oz	200
Sharp, Singles Pasteurized Process Cheese Food (Kraft)	1 oz	150
Smokestick Pasteurized Processed blend of Swiss and Cheddar (Sargento)	1 oz	219
String Cheese—See Mozzarella String Cheese		
Swiss	1 oz	272
Swiss, aged, chunk (Kraft)	1 oz	250
Swiss, aged, slices (Kraft)	1 oz	250
Swiss Almond Nut Log (Sargento)	1 oz	219
Swiss, chunk (Kraft)	1 oz	300
Swiss, Finland (Sargento)	1 oz	272
Swiss, Flavored Pasteurized Process Cheese Product Singles (Light n' Lively)	1 oz	200
Swiss (Land O'Lakes)	1 oz	250
Swiss, Pasteurized Process	1 oz	219
Swiss, Pasteurized Process Cheese Food	1 oz	205
Swiss, Pasteurized Process, slices (Kraft)	1 oz	200

Food	*Portion*	*Calcium (mg)*
Cheese, *continued*		
Swiss, Process Cheese Product, 8% milkfat, slices, Lite-line (Borden)	1 oz	200
Swiss, Process, slices (Borden)	1 oz	350
Swiss (Sargento)	1 oz	272
Swiss, Singles, Pasteurized Process Cheese Food (Kraft)	1 oz	200
Swiss, slices (Kraft)	1 oz	250
Swiss, Spread, Pasteurized Process Cracker Snacks (Sargento)	1 oz	219
Taco blend of Colby and Monterey Jack with taco seasoning (Sargento)	1 oz	203
Tilsit, made with whole milk	1 oz	198
Tilsiter (Sargento)	1 oz	198
Tybo-Red Wax (Sargento)	1 oz	228
CREAM		
Coffee Whitener, nondairy—See Beverages and Juices		
Coffee—See Sweet, Light, Coffee, or Table		
Creamer, imitation, liquid, frozen, made with vegetable fat	1 cup	20
Creamer, imitation, powdered, made with vegetable fat	1 cup	20

Food	Portion	Calcium (mg)
Cream, *continued*		
Half and Half (Land O'Lakes)	1 tbsp.	*
Half and Half, milk and cream	1 tbsp.	16
Half and Half, Sour Cream, cultured	1 tbsp.	16
Half and Half, Sweet Cream, cream and milk	1 cup	254
Half and Half, Sweet Cream, cream and milk	1 tbsp.	16
Ice Cream—See Frozen Dairy Desserts		
Light—See Sweet, Light, Coffee, or Table		
Medium, 25% fat, fluid	1 tbsp.	14
Non-Dairy Creamer (Mrs. Smith's)	1 tbsp.	*
Sour Cream	1 cup	268
Sour Cream, cultured	1 tbsp.	14
Sour Cream (Land O'Lakes)	1 tbsp.	*
Sour, Imitation, nondairy, cultured	1 cup	6
Sweet, Light, Coffee, or Table	1 cup	231
Sweet, Light, Coffee, or Table	1 tbsp.	14
Table—See Sweet, Light, Coffee, or Table		
Topping, Whipped	1 cup	61
Topping, Whipped, powdered, made with whole milk	1 cup	60

**Contains less than 20 milligrams of calcium.*

Food	*Portion*	*Calcium (mg)*
Cream, *continued*		
Whip 'N Top (Mrs. Smith's)	1 tsp	*
Whipped Topping, pressurized	1 cup	61
Whipping, heavy	1 tbsp	10
Whipping, heavy gourmet (Land O'Lakes)	1 tbsp	*
Whipping Cream (Land O'Lakes)	1 tbsp	*
Whipping, light, unwhipped	1 tbsp	10
EGGS		
Chicken Egg, White	1 cup	27
Chicken Egg, Whole	1 egg	28
Chicken Egg, Whole, cooked, fried	1 egg	26
Chicken Egg, Whole, cooked, omelet	1 egg	47
Chicken Egg, Whole, cooked, poached	1 egg	28
Chicken Egg, Whole, cooked, scrambled with butter and milk	1 cup	162
Chicken Egg, Whole, hard-cooked	1 egg	28
Chicken Egg, Yolk	1 cup	368
Duck, Egg, Whole	1 egg	45
Egg Beaters, cholesterol-free egg product (Fleischmann's)	1/4 cup	20
Egg Beaters with Cheez, 99% real egg product (Fleischmann's)	1/2 cup	200
Frozen Breakfasts—See Prepared Main Dishes		

**Contains less than 20 milligrams of calcium.*

Food	*Portion*	*Calcium (mg)*
Eggs, *continued*		
Quiche, Bacon & Onion, Pour-A-Quiche (Land O'Lakes)	$4^1/_3$ oz	300
Quiche, Cheese, Three, Pour-A-Quiche (Land O'Lakes)	$4^1/_3$ oz	300
Quiche, Ham, Pour-A-Quiche (Land O'Lakes)	$4^1/_3$ oz	250
Quiche Mix (Mrs. Smith's)	$^1/_8$ quiche	102
Quiche, Spinach & Onion, Pour-A-Quiche (Land O'Lakes)	$4^1/_3$ oz	300
Substitute, frozen	$^1/_4$ cup	44
Substitute, liquid	1 cup	133
Substitute, powder	0.7 oz	65
MILK		
Acidophilus (Ludwig)	1 cup	300
Butter, regular	1 stick	27
Buttermilk, All Purpose, reconstituted (Swiss Miss)	8 oz	250
Buttermilk, cultured	1 cup	285
Buttermilk, cultured (Borden)	1 cup	300
Buttermilk, fluid, cultured, made from skim milk	1 cup	300
Buttermilk (Land O'Lakes)	8 fl oz	300
Chocolate, 1% (Land O'Lakes)	8 fl oz	300
Chocolate Beverage, Hot Cocoa, prepared with whole milk	1 cup	298

Food	*Portion*	*Calcium (mg)*
Milk, *continued*		
Chocolate drink, fluid, commercial (approximately 90% milk) made with whole milk	1 cup	300
Chocolate drink, same as above, except made with skim milk	1 cup	250
Chocolate (Land O'Lakes)	8 fl oz	300
Chocolate, Lowfat, 1% fat	1 cup	287
Chocolate, Lowfat, 2% fat	1 cup	284
Chocolate, Lowfat, 2% fat (Hershey's)	1 cup	300
Chocolate Milk, Dutch, vitamin D added (Borden)	1 cup	300
Chocolate, skim (Land O'Lakes)	8 fl oz	300
Chocolate, Whole	1 cup	280
Cocoa, hot, homemade with whole milk	1 cup	300
Cocoa, Hot—See Milk, Chocolate Beverage		
Condensed Milk, sweetened (Eagle Brand)	1/3 cup	300
Condensed, sweetened	1 fl oz	108
Condensed, sweetened, canned, concentrated, undiluted	1 cup	800
Dry, Buttermilk	1 tbsp	77
Dry, Nonfat	1/4 cup	377
Dry, Nonfat, instant, reconstituted	1 cup	300
Dry, Nonfat, instantized	1 cup	837

Food	*Portion*	*Calcium (mg)*
Milk, *continued*		
Dry, Nonfat, reconstituted (Carnation)	8 fl oz	279
Dry, Whole	1/4 cup	292
Eggnog	8 fl oz	330
Eggnog (Land O'Lakes)	8 fl oz	300
Evaporated, Carnation	1 fl oz	74
Evaporated, Lowfat (Carnation)	1 fl oz	80
Evaporated, Skim, canned	1 fl oz	92
Evaporated, Skimmed (Carnation)	1 fl oz	92
Evaporated, unsweetened, canned, concentrated, undiluted	1 cup	600
Evaporated, unsweetened, canned, concentrated, undiluted	1 fl oz	80
Evaporated, Whole, canned	1 fl oz	82
Goat	1 cup	326
Homogenized, vitamin D (Borden)	1 cup	300
Human, Whole, mature	1 cup	79
Ice Milk—See Frozen Dairy Desserts		
Imitation, containing blend of hydrogenated vegetable oils	1 cup	79
Lowfat, 1% fat	1 cup	300
Lowfat, 1% (Land O'Lakes)	8 fl oz	300
Lowfat, 2% fat	1 cup	297
Lowfat, 2% fat, protein fortified	1 cup	352
Lowfat, 2% (Land O'Lakes)	8 fl oz	300

Food	Portion	Calcium (mg)
Milk, *continued*		
Lowfat, 2% protein fortified vitamins A and D (Hi-Protein brand/ Borden)	1 cup	350
Lowfat, Chocolate 1%, vitamins A and D added (Dutch Brand/Borden)	1 cup	300
Malted, beverage	1 cup	300
Malted, Chocolate Flavor	2 to 3 heaping tsp	13
Malted, Chocolate Flavor, beverage, with 1 cup milk	3/4 oz powder	304
Malted, Chocolate, instant, with 1 cup milk (Kraft)	3 tsp powder	300
Malted, dry powder, approximately 3 heaping tsp per oz	1 oz	80
Malted, Natural Flavor	2 to 3 heaping tsp	56
Malted, Natural Flavor, beverage with 1 cup milk	3/4 oz powder	347
Malted, Natural, instant (Carnation)	3 heaping tsp	63
Malted, Natural, with 1 cup milk, instant (Kraft)	3 tsp powder	350
Margarine, Corn	1 stick	34
Nonfat Milk, protein fortified, vitamins A and D (Skim-line/Borden)	1 cup	350
Nonfat, Skim	1 cup	300
Shake, Chocolate, thick	10.6 oz	396
Shake, Vanilla, thick	11 oz	457
Skim	1 cup	302
Skim, homogenized, vitamins A and D (Borden)	1 cup	300

Food	*Portion*	*Calcium (mg)*
Milk, *continued*		
Whole, 3.3% fat	1 cup	291
Whole, 3.5% fat	1 cup	300
Whole, homogenized (Land O'Lakes)	1 cup	300
Whole, low sodium	1 cup	246
YOGURT		
Apple, Dutch, Fruit-on-the-Bottom (Dannon)	8 oz	345
Banana & Strawberries (Dannon Supreme)	6 oz	250
Banana, Custard Style (Yoplait)	6 oz	200
Berry, Mixed, Custard Style (Yoplait)	6 oz	200
Blueberry, Fruit-on-the-Bottom (Dannon)	8 oz	345
Cherry (Whitney's)	6 oz	250
Fruit varieties, Lowfat	8 oz.	314
Lemon, Custard Style (Yoplait)	6 oz	200
Orange, Original (Yoplait)	6 oz	250
Peach (Whitney's)	6 oz	250
Plain (Dannon)	8 oz.	415
Plain, Lowfat	8 oz.	415
Raspberry, Fruit-on-the-Bottom (Dannon)	8 oz	345
Strawberry (Whitney's)	6 oz	250
Strawberry-Banana, Original (Yoplait)	6 oz	250
Tropical Fruits Breakfast (Yoplait)	6 oz	200
Vanilla Custard Style Yogurt (Yoplait)	6 oz	250
Vanilla (Dannon)	8 oz	389

FISH AND SHELLFISH

Food	*Portion*	*Calcium (mg)*
FRESH FISH AND SHELLFISH		
Bass, striped, oven-fried	3 oz	20
Clams, raw, meat only	3 oz	59
Cod, broiled, with butter or margarine	3 oz	20
Crabmeat, cooked, steamed	3 oz	40
Flounder, baked, with butter or margarine	3 oz	20
Haddock, breaded, fried	3 oz	34
Halibut, Atlantic and Pacific, broiled, with butter or margarine	3 oz	20
Lobster, northern, cooked	3 oz	60
Mackerel, Atlantic, broiled, with butter or margarine	3 oz	*
Oysters, Eastern, raw, meat only	1 cup	250
Oysters, fried, 4 select (medium), dipped in egg, milk or water, and bread crumbs	1.6 oz	60
Oysters, Pacific, raw meat only, approximately 4–6 medium	1 cup	200
Perch, Ocean, breaded, fried	1 fillet	28

**Contains less than 20 milligrams of calcium.*

Food	*Portion*	*Calcium (mg)*
Fresh Fish and Shellfish, *continued*		
Salmon, smoked	1 oz	*
Salmon steak, broiled or baked, with butter or margarine	3 oz	100
Shrimp, French fried	3 oz	61
Swordfish, broiled, with butter or margarine	3 oz	20
FROZEN FISH AND SHELLFISH		
Clams, Fried, in a light batter (Mrs. Paul's)	2½ oz	*
Crab, Deviled, breaded (Mrs. Paul's)	1 piece	100
Crab, Deviled Miniatures, breaded (Mrs. Paul's)	3½ oz	100
Fish and Chips, Batter-Dipped (Van de Kamp's)	7 oz	50
Fish dinner, frozen—See Prepared Main Dishes		
Fish Fillets, batter dipped (Mrs. Paul's)	2 fillets	20
Fish Fillets, batter, Supreme Light (Mrs. Paul's)	1 fillet	60
Fish Fillets, breaded, Crispy Crunchy (Mrs. Paul's)	2 fillets	20
Fish Fillets, buttered (Mrs. Paul's)	2 fillets	20
Fish Sticks, batter, Crunchy Light (Mrs. Paul's)	4 sticks	20
Fish Sticks, breaded, cooked (4 × 1 × ½ inch)	1 stick or 1 oz	3
Fish Sticks, breaded, Crispy Crunchy (Mrs. Paul's)	4 sticks	20

**Contains less than 20 milligrams of calcium.*

Food	*Portion*	*Calcium (mg)*
Frozen Fish and Shellfish, *continued*		
Flounder, Breaded Lightly (Van de Kamp's)	5 oz	50
Flounder Fillets, batter, Crunchy Light (Mrs. Paul's)	2 fillets	40
Flounder Fillets, breaded, light (Mrs. Paul's)	1 fillet	40
Haddock Fillets, batter, Crunchy Light (Mrs. Paul's)	2 fillets	40
Haddock Fillets, breaded, Crispy Crunchy (Mrs. Paul's)	2 fillets	40
Haddock Fillets, breaded, light (Mrs. Paul's)	1 fillet	40
Perch Fillets, breaded, Crispy Crunchy (Mrs. Paul's)	2 fillets	20
Scallops, breaded, reheated (15–20 per pound)	1 scallop	20
Scallops, French Fried, breaded (Mrs. Paul's)	3½ oz	60
Shrimp, Fried, breaded (Mrs. Paul's)	3 oz	40
Sole, Batter-Dipped (Van de Kamp's)	4 oz	50
Sole, Breaded Lightly (Van de Kamp's)	5 oz	50
Sole Fillets, breaded, light (Mrs. Paul's)	1 fillet	40
CANNED FISH AND SHELLFISH		
Anchovy, pickled, not heavily salted, flat or rolled	5 anchovies	40

Food	*Portion*	*Calcium (mg)*
Canned Fish and Shellfish, *continued*		
Clams, Minced (Snow's)	6 1/2 oz	40
Clams, solids and liquid	3 oz	47
Crabmeat, white or king, not pressed down	1 cup	61
Herring, smoked, kippered fillet (4 3/8 × 1 3/4 × 1/4 inch)	1 fillet	20
Salmon Chum/Keta, with bones (Bumble Bee)	1 cup	548
Salmon, Pink, with bones (Bumble Bee)	1 cup	431
Salmon, Pink (Del Monte)	1/2 cup	200
Salmon, Pink, drained, with bones	3 oz	150
Salmon, Pink, solids and liquid	3 oz	167
Salmon, Red (Del Monte)	1/2 cup	250
Salmon, Red Sockeye, with bones (Bumble Bee)	1 cup	570
Salmon, Red Sockeye, drained, with bones	3 oz	200
Sardines, Atlantic, in oil, drained solids	3 oz	372
Sardines in Tomato Sauce (Del Monte)	1/2 cup	300
Sardines, Smoked Brisling in Olive Oil, drained without liquid (King Oscar)	3 oz	300
Shrimp meat	3 oz	98
Tuna in oil, drained solids	3 oz	7
Tuna in water, solids and liquid	3 oz	*

**Contains less than 20 milligrams of calcium.*

MEAT AND POULTRY

Food	*Portion*	*Calcium (mg)*
BEEF		
Beef, boneless chuck and chuck cuts	1 lb.	59
Beef, corned	1 lb.	41
Beef, dried, chipped, cooked, creamed	1 lb.	476
Beef, dried, chipped, uncooked	1 lb.	91
Beef Meat Pie (Banquet)	8 oz	22
Beef potpie, home prepared, whole (9 inch diameter)	1 pie	88
Beef, Sliced, with Vegetables (Banquet Gourmet)	10 oz	78
Beef Stew (Wolf)	scant cup	34
Beef Tips with Vegetables (Banquet Gourmet)	10 oz	49
Chuck Roast, ground	1 cup	13
Flank Steak	1 lb.	43
Frozen Dinners—See Prepared Main Dishes		
Porterhouse Steak	1 lb.	41
Round Steak	1 lb.	54
Rump Roast	1 lb.	45
Sirloin Steak without bone	1 lb.	45

Food	*Portion*	*Calcium (mg)*
LAMB		
Leg without bone	1 lb.	45
Loin chops	1 lb.	35
Rib chops	1 lb.	33
PORK		
Bacon, cooked	3 medium slices	2
Frozen Dinners—See Prepared Main Dishes		
Ham, Boneless, regular	3 oz	7
Pork, Cured, Canadian-Style Bacon	2 slices	5
Pork Loin, fresh	3 oz	8
VEAL		
Chuck cuts, boneless for stew, without bone	1 lb.	50
Frozen Dinners—See Prepared Main Dishes		
Loin cuts, without bone	1 lb.	50
Round, without bone	1 lb.	50
CHICKEN		
Breast Meat and Skin, Broilers or Fryers, cooked, fried, batter dipped	1/2 breast	28
Breast Meat and Skin, Broilers or Fryers, cooked, fried, flour coated	1/2 breast	16
Breast Meat and Skin, Broilers or Fryers, cooked, roasted	1/2 breast	14
Broilers or Fryers, Flesh and Skin, roasted	1/2 chicken	45
Broilers or Fryers, Flesh and Skin, stewed	1/2 chicken	44

Food	*Portion*	*Calcium (mg)*
Chicken, *continued*		
Broilers or Fryers, Flesh only, fried	1 cup	24
Drumstick Meat and Skin, Broilers or Fryers, cooked, fried, batter dipped	1 drumstick	12
Drumstick Meat and Skin, Broilers or Fryers, cooked, roasted	1 drumstick	6
Frozen Dinners—See Prepared Main Dishes		
Fryers—See Broilers		
Giblets, Broilers or Fryers, cooked, fried, flour coated	1 cup	26
Liver, Broilers or Fryers, simmered	1 cup	20
Liver Pate, canned	1 oz	3
Roasting Dark Meat without Skin, cooked, roasted	1 cup	15
Roasting Flesh and Skin, cooked, roasted	1/2 chicken	58
Roasting Light Meat without Skin, cooked, roasted	1 cup	18
TURKEY		
Breast Fillets with Cheese (Land O' Lakes)	5 oz	150
Breast Meat and Skin, prebasted, roasted	1 breast	149
Breast Meat and Skin, roasted	1/2 breast	182
Dark Meat with Skin, roasted	1/2 turkey	263

Food	*Portion*	*Calcium (mg)*
Turkey, *continued*		
Diced, white/dark mixed (Land O' Lakes)	3 oz	20
Frozen Dinners—See Prepared Main Dishes		
Leg Meat and Skin, roasted	1 leg	176
Light Meat, roasted	1/2 turkey	225
Patties (Land O' Lakes)	2 1/4 oz	40
Roasted	1/2 turkey	488
SAUSAGES, LUNCHEON MEATS, AND SPREADS		
Bologna, Beef	1 oz	3
Bologna, Beef and Pork	1 oz	3
Bologna, Pork	1 oz	3
Bratwurst, Pork, cooked	1 oz	13
Braunschweiger	1 oz	2
Chicken Roll, light meat	1 oz	12
Chicken Spread, canned	1 oz	35
Chicken Spread (Swanson)	1 oz	60
Frankfurter, Beef	2 oz	7
Frankfurter, Beef and Pork	2 oz	6
Frankfurter, Chicken	1 oz	27
Ham Salad Spread	1 tbsp.	1
Ham, sliced	1 slice	2
Kielbasa, Pork, beef, nonfat dry milk added	1 slice	11
Knockwurst	1 link	7
Pastrami, Turkey	2 slices	5
Salami, Beef and Pork, cooked	1 oz	4
Sausage, Italian, Pork, cooked	1 link	16
Sausages, Frozen Breakfasts—See Prepared Main Dishes		
Turkey, Breast Meat	1 slice	1

VEGETABLES

Food	*Portion*	*Calcium (mg)*
ARTICHOKES		
Artichoke, cooked	1 medium	47
Artichoke, frozen, cooked	3 oz	17
Artichoke Hearts, frozen (C&W Frozen Foods)	100 grams	51
ASPARAGUS		
Asparagus, canned	½ cup	17
Asparagus, cooked	½ cup	22
Asparagus, frozen, cooked	10 oz	68
Asparagus, raw	½ cup	14
Asparagus Spears, frozen (C&W Frozen Foods)	100 grams	22
BEAN CURD		
Tofu	½ lb.	290
BEANS		
Bean Salad, Garden, frozen (C&W Frozen Foods)	100 grams	40
Beans & Franks in Tomato & Molasses Sauce (Campbell's)	7⅞ oz	100
Beans, Baked, Brick Oven (B & M)	8 oz	100
Beans and Bacon, (Hormel)	7½ oz.	112
Beans, Green, cut, in Butter Sauce (Green Giant)	½ cup	20

Food	*Portion*	*Calcium (mg)*
Beans, *continued*		
Beans, Green, cut, Kitchen, canned (Green Giant)	½ cup	20
Beans, Green, cut, No Salt Added (Del Monte)	½ cup	20
Beans, Green, French style (Del Monte)	½ cup	20
Beans, Green, French Style, in Butter Sauce (Green Giant)	½ cup	20
Beans, Green, French style, No Salt Added (Del Monte)	½ cup	20
Beans, Italian Cut, frozen (C&W Frozen Foods)	100 grams	35
Beans, Kidney	1 cup	31
Beans, Kidney, Red, Dark, canned (Van Camp's)	8 oz	52
Beans, Lima, cooked	½ cup	27
Beans, Lima, Fordhook, frozen, cooked	½ cup	19
Beans, Lima, Harvest Fresh (Green Giant)	½ cup	20
Beans, Lima, polybag (Green Giant)	½ cup	20
Beans, Mung, sprouted, raw	6 oz	22
Beans, Pinto, frozen, cooked	3⅓ oz	49
Beans, Pork and, canned, in Tomato Sauce (Campbell's)	8 oz	60
Beans, Pork and, canned (Van Camp's)	8 oz	97
Beans, Red, canned (Van Camp's)	8 oz	84

Food	*Portion*	*Calcium (mg)*
Beans, *continued*		
Beans, Refried, Spicy (Del Monte)	½ cup	40
Beans, Snap, canned, solids and liquid	½ cup	29
Beans, Snap, cooked	½ cup	29
Beans, Snap, frozen, cooked	½ cup	31
Beans, Snap, raw	½ cup	21
Beans, Vegetarian Style, canned (Van Camp's)	8 oz	93
Beans, Western Style, canned (Van Camp's)	8 oz	73
Beans, Whole, Petite, frozen (C&W Frozen Foods)	100 grams	40
BEETS		
Beet Greens, cooked	½ cup	82
Beet Greens, raw	½ cup	23
Beets, Harvard, canned, solids and liquid, slices	1 cup	27
Beets, Pickled, canned, solids and liquid, slices	1 cup	25
BROCCOLI		
Broccoli Broccolettes, frozen (C&W Frozen Foods)	100 grams	41
Broccoli Carrot Fanfare, polybag (Green Giant)	½ cup	20
Broccoli, Cauliflower, Carrots, in Butter Sauce (Green Giant)	½ cup	20
Broccoli, Cauliflower, Carrots, in Cheese Flavored Sauce (Green Giant)	½ cup	60

Food	*Portion*	*Calcium (mg)*
Broccoli, *continued*		
Broccoli, Cauliflower Supreme, polybag (Green Giant)	½ cup	20
Broccoli, Cut, Harvest Fresh (Green Giant)	½ cup	20
Broccoli Cuts, polybag (Green Giant)	½ cup	20
Broccoli Fanfare, Harvest Get Togethers (Green Giant)	½ cup	20
Broccoli, fresh, cooked (boiled), drained, chopped	½ cup (78 grams)	89
Broccoli, fresh, raw, chopped	½ cup (44 grams)	21
Broccoli, frozen, cooked (boiled), drained, chopped	½ cup (92 grams)	47
Broccoli, frozen, cooked (boiled), drained, spears	½ cup (92 grams)	47
Broccoli in Cheddar Cheese Sauce (Stouffer's)	4½ oz	150
Broccoli in Cheese Flavored Sauce (Green Giant)	½ cup	60
Broccoli in White Cheddar Cheese Flavored Sauce (Green Giant)	½ cup	60
Broccoli Spears, frozen (C&W Frozen Foods)	100 grams	41
Broccoli Spears, Harvest Fresh (Green Giant)	½ cup	20
Broccoli Spears in Butter Sauce (Green Giant)	½ cup	20
Broccoli with Cheese in Pastry (Pepperidge Farm)	1 pastry	60

Food	*Portion*	*Calcium (mg)*
BRUSSELS SPROUTS		
Brussels Sprouts, Baby, in Cheese Flavored Sauce (Green Giant)	½ cup	60
Brussels Sprouts, cooked	½ cup	28
Brussels Sprouts, frozen, cooked	1 cup	38
Brussels Sprouts in Butter Sauce (Green Giant)	½ cup	20
Brussels Sprouts, Petite, frozen (C&W Frozen Foods)	100 grams	21
Brussels Sprouts, polybag (Green Giant)	½ cup	20
CABBAGE		
Cabbage, Chinese, cooked, shredded	½ cup	79
Cabbage, Chinese, raw, shredded	½ cup	37
Cabbage, cooked, shredded	½ cup	25
Cabbage, raw	1 cup	32
Cabbage, Red, cooked, shredded	½ cup	28
Cabbage, Red, shredded	1 cup	36
CARROTS		
Carrots, Baby, whole, frozen (C&W Frozen Foods)	100 grams	33
Carrots, canned, slices	½ cup	31
Carrots, cooked, slices	½ cup	24
Carrots, frozen, cooked, slices	½ cup	21
Carrots Parisienne, Petite, frozen (C&W Frozen Foods)	100 grams	33
Carrots, raw, shredded	1 cup	30

Food	*Portion*	*Calcium (mg)*
CAULIFLOWER		
Cauliflower and Cheese Sauce in Pastry (Pepperidge Farm)	1 pastry	60
Cauliflower, cooked	1 cup	34
Cauliflower, frozen, cooked	1 cup	30
Cauliflower in Cheese Flavored Sauce (Green Giant)	½ cup	60
Cauliflower in White Cheddar Cheese Flavored Sauce (Green Giant)	½ cup	60
Cauliflower, raw	1 cup	28
CELERY		
Celery, cooked, diced	½ cup	27
Celery, raw, diced	½ cup	22
CHICORY GREENS		
Chicory Greens, raw, chopped	½ cup	90
CHILES		
Chile, Green, whole or diced (Del Monte)	½ cup	60
Chile, Jalapeno, whole or sliced (Del Monte)	½ cup	20
COLLARDS		
Collards, cooked, chopped	½ cup	74
Collards, frozen, chopped	½ cup	179
Collards, raw, chopped	½ cup	109
CORN		
Corn Fritters (2 × 1½ inches)	1 fritter	20
Corn Fritters (Mrs. Paul's)	2 fritters	20
Corn on the Cob, frozen (C&W Frozen Foods)	100 grams	3
Corn Souffle (Stouffer's)	4 oz	40

Food	*Portion*	*Calcium (mg)*
DANDELION GREENS		
Dandelion Greens, cooked, chopped	½ cup	73
Dandelion Greens, raw, chopped	½ cup	52
ENDIVE		
Endive, raw, chopped	1 cup	26
GREENS		
Greens—See Beet Greens, Chicory Greens, Collards, Dandelion Greens, Mustard Greens, Turnip Greens		
KALE		
Kale, cooked, chopped	½ cup	47
Kale, frozen, cooked, chopped	½ cup	90
Kale, raw, chopped	½ cup	46
Kale, Scotch, chopped	½ cup	86
KOHLRABI		
Kohlrabi, cooked, slices	½ cup	20
LEEKS		
Leeks, raw, chopped	½ cup	30
MUSTARD GREENS		
Mustard Greens, cooked, chopped	½ cup	52
Mustard Greens, frozen, cooked, chopped	½ cup	75
Mustard Greens, raw, chopped	½ cup	29
Mustard Spinach, cooked, chopped	½ cup	142
Mustard Spinach, raw, chopped	½ cup	158

Food	*Portion*	*Calcium (mg)*
OKRA		
Okra, cooked, slices	½ cup	50
Okra, frozen, cooked	½ cup	88
Okra, raw, slices	½ cup	41
ONIONS		
Onion Rings, French Fried (Mrs. Paul's)	2¼ oz	20
Onion Rings, frozen, prepared	7 rings	21
Onions, cooked, boiled, chopped	½ cup	29
Onions, raw, chopped	½ cup	20
Onions, small, whole, frozen (C&W Frozen Foods)	100 grams	24
PARSNIPS		
Parsnips, cooked, slices	½ cup	29
Parsnips, raw, slices	½ cup	24
PEAS		
Peas, cooked	½ cup	33
Peas, Early June, canned (Green Giant)	½ cup	20
Peas, Sweet, No Salt Added (Del Monte)	½ cup	20
POTATOES		
Potato Salad	1 cup	80
Potatoes Au Gratin	½ cup	146
Potatoes, baked	1 potato	20
Potatoes, mashed, flakes (Hungry Jack), with added ingredients	½ cup	40
Potatoes, mashed, milk and butter added	1 cup	40
Potatoes, mashed, Potato Buds (Betty Crocker), with added ingredients	⅓ cup buds	20

Food	*Portion*	*Calcium (mg)*
PUMPKIN		
Pumpkin, cooked, mashed	1 cup	37
Pumpkin (Del Monte)	½ cup	20
Pumpkin Pie Mix, canned	½ cup	49
SAUERKRAUT		
Sauerkraut, canned	½ cup	36
Sauerkraut (Del Monte)	½ cup	20
SPINACH		
Spinach, chopped, frozen (C&W Frozen Foods)	100 grams	113
Spinach, chopped or whole, leaf (Del Monte)	½ cup	100
Spinach, cooked	½ cup	122
Spinach, Creamed (Green Giant)	½ cup	100
Spinach, Creamed (Stouffer's)	4½ oz	100
Spinach, frozen	1 cup	173
Spinach, Harvest Fresh (Green Giant)	½ cup	100
Spinach, Leaf, frozen (C&W Frozen Foods)	100 grams	105
Spinach, New Zealand, cooked, chopped	1 cup	86
Spinach, New Zealand, raw, chopped	1 cup	32
Spinach, raw, chopped	½ cup	28
Spinach Souffle (Stouffer's)	4 oz	80
Spinach, whole leaf, No Salt Added (Del Monte)	½ cup	100
SQUASH		
Squash, Acorn, cooked	1 cup	90
Squash, Acorn, mashed	1 cup	65
Squash, Butternut, cooked	1 cup	84
Squash, Butternut, frozen, mashed	1 cup	45

Food	Portion	Calcium (mg)
SWEET POTATOES		
Sweet Potatoes, baked in skin, mashed	½ cup	28
Sweet Potatoes, canned	1 cup	44
SWISS CHARD		
Swiss Chard	1 leaf	24
Swiss Chard, cooked, chopped	½ cup	51
Swiss Chard, frozen (C&W Frozen Foods)	100 grams	73
TOMATOES		
Tomato Paste, canned	½ cup	46
Tomato Paste (Contadina)	6 oz	48
Tomato Paste (Del Monte)	¾ cup	60
Tomato Paste (Hunt's)	2 oz	20
Tomato Paste Italian Style (Hunt's)	2 oz	20
Tomato Paste, No Salt Added (Del Monte)	6 oz	60
Tomato Paste, No Salt Added (Hunt's)	2 oz	20
Tomato Puree, canned	1 cup	37
Tomato Puree (Hunt's)	4 oz	20
Tomato Sauce, canned	1 cup	34
Tomato Sauce, Spanish style, canned	½ cup	20
Tomato Sauce—See Also Sauces		
Tomatoes, Baby, sliced (Contadina)	½ cup	83
Tomatoes, Italian style (Contadina)	½ cup	20
Tomatoes, Red, canned	½ cup	32
Tomatoes, Red, chopped	1 cup	12
Tomatoes, Red, cooked	1 cup	20

Food	Portion	Calcium (mg)
Tomatoes, *continued*		
Tomatoes, Stewed (Contadina)	½ cup	40
Tomatoes, Stewed (Del Monte)	½ cup	20
Tomatoes, Stewed (Hunt's)	4 oz	40
Tomatoes, Stewed, No Salt Added (Del Monte)	½ cup	20
Tomatoes, Stewed, No Salt Added (Hunt's)	4 oz	40
Tomatoes, wedges (Del Monte)	½ cup	20
Tomatoes, whole (Hunt's)	4 oz	40
Tomatoes, whole, peeled (Contadina)	½ cup	40
Tomatoes, whole, peeled (Del Monte)	½ cup	20
TURNIPS		
Turnip Greens, cooked, chopped	½ cup	99
Turnip Greens, frozen	½ cup	125
Turnips, cooked, mashed	½ cup	26
Turnips, raw, cubed	½ cup	20
YAMS		
Yam, cooked, cubed	1 cup	19
Yams and Apples (Stouffer's)	5 oz	20
Yams, Candied, 'n' Apples (Mrs. Paul's)	4 oz	40
ZUCCHINI		
Zucchini in Tomato Sauce (Del Monte)	½ cup	20
Zucchini, raw, slices	1 cup	20
Zucchini Sticks, Light Batter (Mrs. Paul's)	3 oz	20

FRUITS

Food	*Portion*	*Calcium (mg)*
APPLES		
Apple Fritters (Mrs. Paul's)	2 fritters	80
Apple Juice—See Beverages and Juices		
Apples, raw, with skin	1 fruit	10
Applesauce, canned, sweetened	1 cup	9
APRICOTS		
Apricots, canned, heavy syrup, whole	1 cup	22
Apricots, canned, juice pack, halves	1 cup	30
Apricots, canned, water pack, halves	1 cup	19
Apricots, dried, sulfured, uncooked, halves	1 cup	59
Apricots, raw, halves	1 cup	22
Apricots, uncooked, dried (Del Monte)	2 oz	20
AVOCADOS		
Avocados	1 fruit	22
BANANAS		
Bananas	1 fruit	7
BLACKBERRIES		
Blackberries, canned, heavy syrup	½ cup	27
Blackberries, frozen, unsweetened	1 cup	44

Food	*Portion*	*Calcium (mg)*
BOYSENBERRIES		
Boysenberries, canned, heavy syrup	½ cup	23
Boysenberries, frozen, unsweetened	1 cup	36
CANTALOUPE		
Cantaloupe	½ melon	28
CHERRIES		
Cherries, Sour Red, canned	1 cup	26
Cherries, Sour Red, without pits	1 cup	24
Cherries, Sweet, canned	1 cup	27
Cherries, Sweet, frozen, sweetened	1 cup	31
Cherries, Sweet, raw	1 cup	21
CRANBERRIES		
Cranberries, raw, chopped	1 cup	8
Cranberry Juice, bottled—See Beverages and Juices		
Cranberry-Orange Relish, canned	1 cup	29
Cranberry Sauce, canned, sweetened	1 cup	10
CURRANTS		
Currants, European Black	½ cup	31
Currants, Zante (Del Monte)	½ cup	60
DATES		
Dates, chopped	1 cup	58
Dates, chopped (Dromedary)	¼ cup	20
Dates, pitted (Dromedary)	5 dates	20
FIGS		
Figs, raw	1 large	22
Figs, whole, canned (Del Monte)	½ cup	20

Food	*Portion*	*Calcium (mg)*
FRUIT COCKTAIL		
Fruit Cocktail, canned, in heavy syrup, fruit and liquid	1 cup	20
Fruit Cocktail, canned, juice pack	1 cup	20
FRUIT SALAD		
Fruit Salad, canned, juice pack	1 cup	28
Fruit Salad, Tropical, canned	1 cup	34
GRAPEFRUIT		
Grapefruit, canned	1 cup	37
Grapefruit Juice—See Beverages and Juices		
Grapefruit; raw; pink, red, and white sections, with juice	1 cup	27
GRAPES		
Grape Juice—See Beverages and Juices		
Grapes	1 cup	17
Grapes, canned	1 cup	25
KIWIFRUIT		
Kiwifruit	1 large	24
LEMONS		
Lemons, raw, without peel	1 large	22
LIMES		
Limes	1 fruit	22
MELON		
Melon Balls, Mixed, frozen (C&W Frozen Foods)	100 grams	12
Melons—See Cantaloupe and Watermelon		

Food	*Portion*	*Calcium (mg)*
ORANGES		
Orange Juice—See Beverages and Juices		
Oranges	1 fruit	52
PAPAYAS		
Papayas	1 fruit	72
PEACHES		
Peaches	1 fruit	5
Peaches, canned, juice pack, halves or slices	1 cup	15
Peaches, dehydrated, low moisture, sulfured	½ cup	22
Peaches, sliced, frozen (C&W Frozen Foods)	100 grams	6
PEARS		
Pears	1 fruit	19
Pears, canned, halves	1 cup	13
PINEAPPLE		
Pineapple, canned, juice pack, chunks or tidbits	1 cup	34
Pineapple, diced, pieces	1 cup	11
Pineapple, fresh (Del Monte)	½ cup	20
Pineapple Juice—See Beverages and Juices		
Pineapple Spears, in juice, canned (Del Monte)	2 spears	20
PLUMS		
Plums	1 plum............	2
Plums, Purple, canned, juice pack	1 cup	25
PRUNES		
Prune Juice—See Beverages and Juices		
Prunes, canned	1 cup	40

Food	Portion	Calcium (mg)
PRUNES, *continued*		
Prunes, dried, uncooked	1 cup	82
Prunes, Moist-Pak, dried (Del Monte)	2 oz	20
Prunes, uncooked, pitted, dried (Del Monte)	2 oz	20
Prunes, uncooked, with pits, dried (Del Monte)	2 oz	20
RAISINS		
Raisins, Golden, dried (Del Monte)	3 oz	40
Raisins, Golden, seedless, packed	1 cup	87
Raisins, Natural, dried (Del Monte)	3 oz	40
Raisins, seedless, packed	1 cup	81
RASPBERRIES		
Raspberries	1 cup	27
Raspberries, canned	1 cup	27
RHUBARB		
Rhubarb, diced, pieces	½ cup	52
Rhubarb, frozen, cooked, with added sugar	½ cup	174
STRAWBERRIES		
Strawberries	1 cup	21
Strawberries, canned	½ cup	16
Strawberries, frozen, unsweetened	1 cup	23
TANGELO		
Tangelo, raw, medium (2 9/16 inch diameter)	1 fruit	20
TANGERINES		
Tangerines	1 fruit	12
WATERMELON		
Watermelon	1/16 melon	38

BREADS

Food	*Portion*	*Calcium (mg)*
BREADS		
Banana Quick Bread Mix (Duncan Hines), with added ingredients	one ½ inch slice....	20
Blueberry Nut Quick Bread Mix (Pillsbury), with added ingredients	1/12 loaf	20
Boston Brown Bread, canned (3 ¼ by ½ inch thick)	1 piece	41
Bran, Honey (Pepperidge Farm)	2 slices............	20
Bran, Whole (Brownberry Ovens)	2 slices............	20
Bread Crumbs, toasted, regular style (Old London)	2 oz	60
Carrot Nut Quick Bread Mix (Duncan Hines), with added ingredients	one ½ inch slice....	20
Carrot Nut Quick Bread Mix (Pillsbury), with added ingredients	1/12 loaf	20
Cinnamon (Pepperidge Farm)	2 slices............	20

Food	Portion	Calcium (mg)
Breads, *continued*		
Corn Bread, Easy Mix (Aunt Jemima), with added ingredients	1/6 corn bread	20
Corn Bread Mix, prepared (Dromedary)	2 inches × 2 inches	60
Croutons, Cheese and Garlic (Pepperidge Farm)	1/2 oz	20
Croutons, seasoned (Pepperidge Farm)	1/2 oz	20
Dark (Hollywood)	1 slice	40
Dark Sandwich (Brownberry Ovens)	2 slices	20
French (5 × 2 1/2 × 1 inches)	1 slice	15
French Parisian (DiCarlo)	1 slice	40
French Toast—See Pancakes and Waffles		
French (Wonder)	1 slice	40
Health Nut (Brownberry Ovens)	2 slices	20
Italian, Family (Wonder)	1 slice	40
Light (Hollywood)	1 slice	40
Nut Quick Bread Mix (Duncan Hines), with added ingredients	one 1/2 inch slice	20
Pumpernickel, Family (Pepperidge Farm)	2 slices	40
Raisin (3 3/4 × 3 5/8 × 1/2 inches, 1/18 of loaf)	1 slice	18
Raisin Cinnamon (Brownberry Ovens)	2 slices	20
Raisin Nut (Brownberry Ovens)	2 slices	20
Raisin (Sun-Maid)	1 slice	20
Raisin with Cinnamon (Pepperidge Farm)	2 slices	20

Food	Portion	Calcium (mg)
Breads, *continued*		
Roman Meal	1 slice	40
Rye, Extra Thin (Brownberry Ovens)	2 slices	*
Rye, Family (Pepperidge Farm)	2 slices	40
Rye, seedless (Pepperidge Farm)	2 slices	40
Seven Grain (Home Pride)	1 slice	20
Sour Dough (DiCarlo)	1 slice	20
Stuffing, Chicken Flavored (Banquet)	4 oz	65
Stuffing, Chicken, Stuffing Originals (Green Giant)	½ cup	20
Stuffing, Corn Bread (Pepperidge Farm)	1 oz	20
Stuffing, Cube (Pepperidge Farm)	1 oz	20
Stuffing, Herb Seasoned (Pepperidge Farm)	1 oz	40
Stuffing, Mushroom, Stuffing Originals (Green Giant)	½ cup	20
Vienna (4¾ × 4½ inches)	1 slice	11
Wheatberry (Home Pride)	1 slice	40
Wheat, Butter Top (Home Pride)	1 slice	40
Wheat, Cracked (4 × 4¼ × 9/16 inches)	1 slice	22
Wheat, Cracked (Pepperidge Farm)	2 slices	20
Wheat, Cracked (Wonder)	1 slice	40
Wheat, Family (Wonder)	1 slice	40
Wheat (Fresh Horizons)	1 slice	40

**Contains less than 20 milligrams of calcium.*

Food	Portion	Calcium (mg)
Breads, *continued*		
Wheat, Natural (Brownberry Ovens)	2 slices	20
Wheat, 100% Whole, Soft (Wonder)	1 slice	20
Wheat, Whole (Pepperidge Farm)	2 slices	40
Wheat, Whole, Very Thin (Pepperidge Farm)	2 slices	20
White, Butter Top (Home Pride)	1 slice	40
White, Enriched, Sandwich (Brownberry Ovens)	2 slices	20
White (Fresh Horizons)	1 slice	40
White (Pepperidge Farm)	2 slices	40
White, with Buttermilk (Wonder)	1 slice	40
White (Wonder)	1 slice	40
Zwieback (approximately 3½×1½×½ inches)	1 piece	*
ROLLS		
Bagel, Egg (3 inch diameter)	1 bagel	*
Bagel, Poppy Seed (Sara Lee)	1 bagel	20
Brown 'n Serve, Home Bake (Wonder)	1 roll	40
Brown 'n Serve with Buttermilk (Wonder)	1 roll	40
Club, Brown 'n Serve (Pepperidge Farm)	1 roll	40
Crescent, Butter (Pepperidge Farm)	1 roll	20
Dinner (Home Pride)	1 roll	40

**Contains less than 20 milligrams of calcium.*

Food	Portion	Calcium (mg)
Rolls, *continued*		
Dinner (Wonder)	1 roll	40
Frankfurter or Hamburger enriched	1 roll	20
French Style (Pepperidge Farm)	1 roll	40
Golden Twist (Pepperidge Farm)	1 roll	20
Hamburger Buns (Wonder)	1 bun	40
Hamburger (Pepperidge Farm)	1 roll	40
Hoagie or Submarine (11½ ×3×2½ inches)	1 roll	60
Hoagie (Wonder)	1 roll	200
Hot Dog (Wonder)	1 roll	40
Onion Sandwich Buns with Poppy Seeds (Pepperidge Farm)	1 roll	40
Pan (Wonder)	1 roll	40
Parker House (Pepperidge Farm)	1 roll	20
Sandwich, with Sesame Seeds (Pepperidge Farm)	1 roll	40
Sourdough Style, French (Pepperidge Farm)	1 roll	20
MUFFINS		
Apple Cinnamon Mix (Betty Crocker), with added ingredients	1/12 pkg	20
Apple with Spice, Old Fashioned (Pepperidge Farm)	1 muffin	40
Blueberry, Old Fashioned (Pepperidge Farm)	1 muffin	20
English (Wonder)	1 muffin	150

CEREALS, GRAINS, AND RICE

Food	*Portion*	*Calcium (mg)*
CEREALS		
All-Bran (Kellogg's), with 1/2 cup milk	1 oz cereal	175
All-Bran (Kellogg's), without milk	1 oz	25
All-Bran with Extra Fiber (Kellogg's), with 1/2 cup milk	1 oz cereal	181
All-Bran with Extra Fiber (Kellogg's), without milk	1 oz	31
Apple-Jacks (Kellogg's), with 1/2 cup milk	1 oz cereal	153
Apple-Jacks (Kellogg's), without milk	1 oz	3
Apple Raisin Crisp (Kellogg's), with 1/2 cup milk	1.4 oz cereal	156
Apple Raisin Crisp (Kellogg's), without milk	1.4 oz	6
Body Buddies, Brown Sugar & Honey (General Mills), with 1/2 cup milk	1 oz cereal	250
Body Buddies, Brown Sugar & Honey (General Mills), without milk	1 oz	100

Food	Portion	Calcium (mg)
Cereals, *continued*		
Body Buddies, Natural Fruit Flavor (General Mills), with 1/2 cup milk	1 oz cereal	250
Body Buddies, Natural Fruit Flavor (General Mills), without milk	1 oz	100
BooBerry (General Mills), with 1/2 cup milk	1 oz cereal	170
BooBerry (General Mills), without milk	1 oz	20
Bran-Buds (Kellogg's), with 1/2 cup milk	1 oz cereal	170
Bran-Buds (Kellogg's), without milk	1 oz	20
Bran Flakes (Kellogg's), with 1/2 cup milk	1 oz cereal	163
Bran Flakes (Kellogg's), without milk	1 oz	13
Bran Muffin Crisp (General Mills), with 1/2 cup milk	1.4 oz cereal	210
Bran Muffin Crisp (General Mills), without milk	1.4 oz	60
BucWheats (General Mills), with 1/2 cup milk	1 oz cereal	210
BucWheats (General Mills), without milk	1 oz	60
C-3PO's (Kellogg's), with 1/2 cup milk	1 oz cereal	156
C-3PO's (Kellogg's), without milk	1 oz	6
Cheerios (General Mills), with 1/2 cup milk	1 oz cereal	190

Food	*Portion*	*Calcium (mg)*
Cereals, *continued*		
Cheerios (General Mills), without milk	1 oz	40
Cheerios, Honey Nut (General Mills), with 1/2 cup milk	1 oz cereal	170
Cheerios, Honey Nut (General Mills), without milk	1 oz	20
Cinnamon Toast Crunch (General Mills), with 1/2 cup milk	1 oz cereal	190
Cinnamon Toast Crunch (General Mills), without milk	1 oz	40
Cocoa Krispies (Kellogg's), with 1/2 cup milk	1 oz cereal	156
Cocoa Krispies (Kellogg's), without milk	1 oz	6
Cocoa Puffs (General Mills), with 1/2 cup milk	1 oz cereal	150
Cocoa Puffs (General Mills), without milk	1 oz	*
Corn Flakes, Country (General Mills), with 1/2 cup milk	1 oz cereal	150
Corn Flakes, Country (General Mills), without milk	1 oz	*
Corn Flakes, Honey & Nut (Kellogg's), with 1/2 cup milk	1 oz cereal	154
Corn Flakes, Honey & Nut (Kellogg's), without milk	1 oz	4

**Contains less than 20 milligrams of calcium.*

Food	*Portion*	*Calcium (mg)*
Cereals, *continued*		
Corn Flakes (Kellogg's), with 1/2 cup milk	1 oz cereal	151
Corn Flakes (Kellogg's), without milk	1 oz	1
Corn Grits	1 cup	3
Corn Pops (Kellogg's), with 1/2 cup milk	1 oz cereal	152
Corn Pops (Kellogg's), without milk	1 oz	2
Count Chocula (General Mills), with 1/2 cup milk	1 oz cereal	170
Count Chocula (General Mills), without milk	1 oz	20
Cracklin' Oat Bran (Kellogg's), with 1/2 cup milk	1 oz cereal	169
Cracklin' Oat Bran (Kellogg's), without milk	1 oz	19
Crispix (Kellogg's), with 1/2 cup milk	1 oz cereal	154
Crispix (Kellogg's), without milk	1 oz	4
Crispy Wheats 'n Raisins (General Mills), with 1/2 cup milk	1 oz cereal	190
Crispy Wheats 'n Raisins (General Mills), without milk	1 oz	40
E.T. (General Mills), with 1/2 cup milk	1 oz cereal	150
E.T. (General Mills), without milk	1 oz	*

**Contains less than 20 milligrams of calcium.*

Food	*Portion*	*Calcium (mg)*
Cereals, *continued*		
Fiber One (General Mills) with 1/2 cup milk	1 oz cereal	210
Fiber One (General Mills), without milk	1 oz	60
Frosted Flakes (Kellogg's), with 1/2 cup milk	1 oz cereal	151
Frosted Flakes (Kellogg's), without milk	1 oz	1
Frosted Krispies (Kellogg's), with 1/2 cup milk	1 oz cereal	152
Frosted Krispies (Kellogg's), without milk	1 oz	2
Frosted Mini-Wheats (Kellogg's), with 1/2 cup milk	1 oz cereal	160
Frosted Mini-Wheats (Kellogg's), without milk	1 oz	10
Fruitful Bran (Kellogg's), with 1/2 cup milk	1.3 oz cereal	162
Fruitful Bran (Kellogg's), without milk	1.3 oz	12
Golden Grahams (General Mills), with 1/2 cup milk	1 oz cereal	150
Golden Grahams (General Mills), without milk	1 oz	*
Granola, Cinnamon & Raisin (Nature Valley), with 1/2 cup milk	1 oz granola	150
Granola, Cinnamon & Raisin (Nature Valley), without milk	1 oz	*
Granola, Coconut & Honey (Nature Valley), with 1/2 cup milk	1 oz granola	170

**Contains less than 20 milligrams of calcium.*

Food	Portion	Calcium (mg)
Cereals, *continued*		
Granola, Coconut & Honey (Nature Valley), without milk	1 oz	20
Granola, Fruit & Nut (Nature Valley), with 1/2 cup milk	1 oz granola	170
Granola, Fruit & Nut (Nature Valley), without milk	1 oz	20
Granola, homemade	1 cup	76
Granola, Toasted Oat Mixture (Nature Valley), with 1/2 cup milk	1 oz granola	150
Granola, Toasted Oat Mixture (Nature Valley), without milk	1 oz	*
Kix (General Mills), with 1/2 cup milk	1 oz cereal	190
Kix (General Mills), without milk	1 oz	40
Life, Cinnamon, ready-to-eat (Quaker)	2/3 cup	60
Life, Raisin, ready-to-eat (Quaker)	2/3 cup	60
Life, ready-to-eat (Quaker)	2/3 cup	60
Lucky Charms (General Mills), with 1/2 cup milk	1 oz cereal	170
Lucky Charms (General Mills), without milk	1 oz	20
Marshmallow Krispies (Kellogg's), with 1/2 cup milk	1.3 oz cereal	153
Marshmallow Krispies (Kellogg's), without milk	1.3 oz	3

**Contains less than 20 milligrams of calcium.*

Food	*Portion*	*Calcium (mg)*
Cereals, *continued*		
Nutri·Grain Corn (Kellogg's), with 1/2 cup milk	1 oz cereal	151
Nutri·Grain Corn (Kellogg's), without milk	1 oz	1
Nutri·Grain Wheat & Raisins (Kellogg's), with 1/2 cup milk	1.4 oz cereal	163
Nutri·Grain Wheat & Raisins (Kellogg's), without milk	1.4 oz	13
Nutri·Grain Wheat (Kellogg's), with 1/2 cup milk	1 oz cereal	159
Nutri·Grain Wheat (Kellogg's), without milk	1 oz	9
Oat Bran (Quaker)	1 oz	20
Oat Flakes, Fortified	1 cup	68
Oatmeal, Peaches and Cream Flavor, artificial, instant (Quaker)	1 packet	100
Oatmeal, Regular Flavor, instant (Quaker)	1 packet	100
Oatmeal, Strawberries and Cream Flavor, artificial, instant (Quaker)	1 packet	100
Oatmeal with Apples, Real, and Cinnamon, instant (Quaker)	1 packet	100
Oatmeal with Bran and Raisins, instant (Quaker)	1 packet	100
Oatmeal with Cinnamon and Spice, instant (Quaker)	1 packet	100

Food	*Portion*	*Calcium (mg)*
Cereals, *continued*		
Oatmeal with Honey, Real, and Graham, instant (Quaker)	1 packet	100
Oatmeal with Maple & Brown Sugar Flavors, artificial, instant (Quaker)	1 packet	100
Oatmeal with Raisins and Spice, instant (Quaker)	1 packet	100
Oatmeal with Raisins, Dates, and Walnuts, instant (Quaker)	1 packet	100
Oats, regular, quick, and instant, nonfortified, cooked	1 cup	20
OJ's (Kellogg's), with 1/2 cup milk	1 oz cereal	150
OJ's (Kellogg's), without milk	1 oz	*
Pac-Man (General Mills), with 1/2 cup milk	1 oz cereal	170
Pac-Man (General Mills), without milk	1 oz	20
Product 19 (Kellogg's), with 1/2 cup milk	1 oz cereal	154
Product 19 (Kellogg's), without milk	1 oz	4
Raisin Bran (Kellogg's), with 1/2 cup milk	1.4 oz cereal	163
Raisin Bran (Kellogg's), without milk	1.4 oz	13
Raisin Squares (Kellogg's), with 1/2 cup milk	1 oz cereal	164

*Contains less than 20 milligrams of calcium.

Food	*Portion*	*Calcium (mg)*
Cereals, *continued*		
Raisin Squares (Kellogg's), without milk	1 oz	14
Raisins, Rice, & Rye (Kellogg's), with 1/2 cup milk	1.3 oz cereal	159
Raisins, Rice, & Rye (Kellogg's), without milk	1.3 oz	9
Rice, Cream of, with 2 oz whole milk (Nabisco)	1 oz cereal	80
Rice Krispies (Kellogg's), with 1/2 cup milk	1 oz cereal	153
Rice Krispies (Kellogg's), without milk	1 oz	3
Rice, Puffed	1 cup	1
S'mores Crunch (General Mills), with 1/2 cup milk	1 oz	150
S'mores Crunch (General Mills), without milk	1 oz	*
Special K (Kellogg's), with 1/2 cup milk	1 oz cereal	160
Special K (Kellogg's), without milk	1 oz	10
Strawberry Shortcake (General Mills), with 1/2 cup milk	1 oz cereal	150
Strawberry Shortcake (General Mills), without milk	1 oz	*
Sugar Sparkled Flakes	1 oz	4
Total, Corn (General Mills), with 1/2 cup milk	1 oz cereal	190
Total, Corn (General Mills), without milk	1 oz	40

**Contains less than 20 milligrams of calcium.*

Food	*Portion*	*Calcium (mg)*
Cereals, *continued*		
Total (General Mills), with 1/2 cup milk	1 oz cereal	190
Total (General Mills), without milk	1 oz	40
Trix (General Mills), with 1/2 cup milk	1 oz cereal	150
Trix (General Mills), without milk	1 oz	*
Wheat, Cream of, Apple and Cinnamon, Mix 'n Eat (Nabisco)	1 1/4 oz	40
Wheat, Cream of, Apple and Cinnamon, with 2 oz whole milk, Mix 'n Eat (Nabisco)	1 1/4 oz cereal	115
Wheat, Cream of, Brown Sugar Cinnamon, Mix 'n Eat (Nabisco)	1 1/4 oz	40
Wheat, Cream of, Brown Sugar Cinnamon, with 2 oz whole milk, Mix 'n Eat (Nabisco)	1 1/4 oz cereal	115
Wheat, Cream of, Instant (Nabisco)	1 oz	150
Wheat, Cream of, Instant, with 2 oz whole milk (Nabisco)	1 oz cereal	225
Wheat, Cream of, Maple Brown Sugar, Mix 'n Eat (Nabisco)	1 1/4 oz	40
Wheat, Cream of, Maple Brown Sugar, with 2 oz whole milk, Mix 'n Eat (Nabisco)	1 1/4 oz cereal	115

**Contains less than 20 milligrams of calcium.*

Food	*Portion*	*Calcium (mg)*
Cereals, *continued*		
Wheat, Cream of, Our Original Mix 'n Eat (Nabisco)	1 oz	40
Wheat, Cream of, Our Original, with 2 oz whole milk, Mix 'n Eat (Nabisco)	1 oz cereal	115
Wheat, Cream of, Quick (Nabisco)	1 oz	40
Wheat, Cream of, Quick, with 2 oz whole milk (Nabisco)	1 oz cereal	115
Wheat, Cream of, Regular (Nabisco)	1 oz	40
Wheat, Cream of, Regular, with 2 oz whole milk (Nabisco)	1 oz cereal	115
Wheat, Cream of, Strawberry, Mix 'n Eat (Nabisco)	1¼ oz	40
Wheat, Cream of, Strawberry, with 2 oz whole milk, Mix 'n Eat (Nabisco)	1¼ oz cereal	115
Wheat, Puffed, plain	1 cup	3
Wheat, Shredded, large biscuit	1 biscuit	10
Wheat, Shredded, small biscuit	1 oz	11
Wheaties (General Mills), with ½ cup milk	1 oz cereal	190
Wheaties (General Mills), without milk	1 oz	40

Food	*Portion*	*Calcium (mg)*
GRAINS		
Baking Powder (sodium aluminum sulfate with monocalcium phosphate monohydrate)†	1 tbsp	213
Corn Meal, White Buttermilk Mix, self-rising (Aunt Jemima)	3 tbsp	60
Corn Meal, White Mix, bolted (Aunt Jemima/ Quaker)	1/6 cup	60
Corn Meal, White, self-rising (Aunt Jemima/ Quaker)	1/6 cup	109
Corn Meal, White, self-rising, enriched, bolted (Aunt Jemima/Quaker)	1/6 cup	109
Corn Meal, Yellow Mix, bolted (Aunt Jemima/ Quaker)	1/6 cup	60
De Maiz Masa Harina (Quaker)	1/3 cup	77
Flour, all-purpose (Gold Medal)	4 oz	200
Flour, all-purpose (White Deer)	4 oz	20
Flour, high protein, Better for Bread (Gold Medal)	4 oz	20
Flour, Rye and Wheat, Bohemian Style (Pillsbury's Best)	1 cup	20
Flour, Rye, Medium (Pillsbury's Best)	1 cup	20

†Baking Powder is not a grain, but is generally used in conjunction with grains.

Food	Portion	Calcium (mg)
Grains, *continued*		
Flour, self-rising, enriched (Aunt Jemima/Quaker)	1/4 cup	60
Flour, self-rising (Gold Medal)	4 oz	350
Flour, self-rising (Red Star)	4 oz	200
Flour, Self-Rising, Unbleached or Bleached (Pillsbury's Best and Ballard)	1 cup	300
Flour (Softasilk)	4 oz	*
Flour, unbleached (Gold Medal)	4 oz	20
Flour, Wheat, Whole (Gold Medal)	4 oz	20
Flour, Wheat, Whole (Pillsbury's Best)	1 cup	20
RICE		
Beef flavor Rice & Sauce (Lipton), with added ingredients	1/2 cup	*
Beef flavor Rice-A-Roni, prepared	1.3 oz	40
Chicken flavor Rice & Sauce (Lipton), with added ingredients	1/2 cup	*
Fried Rice, Shrimp (Green Giant)	10 oz	50
Herb & Butter Rice & Sauce (Lipton), with added ingredients	1/2 cup	*
Spanish Rice (Lipton)	1 cup	*
Spanish Rice (Van Camp's)	1 cup	35
Vegetable Rice with Butter (Banquet)	4 oz	20

**Contains less than 20 milligrams of calcium.*

NOODLES AND PASTA

Food	*Portion*	*Calcium (mg)*
Alfredo Noodles & Sauce, Deluxe (Lipton), with added ingredients	½ cup	100
Beef flavor Noodles & Sauce (Lipton), with added ingredients	½ cup	*
Butter & Herb Noodles & Sauce (Lipton), with		
Butter Noodles & Sauce (Lipton), with added ingredients	½ cup	*
Cheese Noodles & Sauce (Lipton), with added ingredients	½ cup	40
Chicken Bombay Noodles & Sauce, Deluxe (Lipton), with added ingredients	½ cup	40
Creamy Garlic Shells & Sauce (Lipton), with added ingredients	½ cup	40
Egg Noodle and Cheese Dinner (Kraft)	¾ cup	100
Egg Noodles (Creamette)	2 oz dry	20

**Contains less than 20 milligrams of calcium.*

Food	*Portion*	*Calcium (mg)*
Egg Noodles (Pennsylvania Dutch Brand), all kinds	2 oz	*
Egg Noodle with Chicken Dinner (Kraft)	3/4 cup	40
Fettuccine Alfredo International Noodle Mix (Betty Crocker), with added ingredients	1/4 pkg	100
Fettucini Alfredo (Stouffer's)	5 oz	150
Frozen Dinners—See Also Prepared Main Dishes		
Lasagna, Dinner Classics (Armour)	1 dinner	200
Lasagna Florentine (Light and Elegant Entrees/ Banquet)	11.25 oz	280
Lasagna frozen dinner (Swanson)	1 dinner	150
Lasagna (Hormel)	7 1/2 oz	41
Lasagna, Sausage, Italian, frozen (Van de Kamp's)	11 oz	450
Lasagna (Stouffer's)	10 1/2 oz	250
Lasagna, Vegetable, frozen dinner (Le Menu/ Swanson)	1 dinner	200
Lasagna Vegetable (Stouffer's)	10 1/2 oz	500
Lasagna with Meat and Sauce (Green Giant) 10.5 oz	1 dinner	450
Lasagna with Meat and Sauce (Green Giant) 12 oz	1 dinner	500

Contains less than 20 milligrams of calcium.

Food	*Portion*	*Calcium (mg)*
Lasagna with Meat, frozen dinner, Hungry-Man (Swanson)	1 dinner	300
Lasagna with Meat Sauce, Family Entree (Banquet)	8 oz	255
Macaroni & Cheese, Elbow (Franco-American)	7⅜ oz	80
Macaroni & Cheese (Franco-American)	7⅜ oz	80
Macaroni and Cheese Dinner (Creamettes)	2 oz	100
Macaroni and Cheese Dinner (Kraft)	¾ cup	80
Macaroni and Cheese (Green Giant)	9 oz	200
Noodles 'n Beef (Hormel)	7½ oz	68
Noodles and Chicken (Dinty Moore)	7½ oz	44
Noodles Chow Mein, canned	1 cup	*
Noodle Dinners—See Also Prepared Main Dishes		
Noodles, Egg, enriched, cooked	1 cup	16
Noodles Romanoff (Stouffer's)	4 oz	60
Parmesano Noodles & Sauce, Deluxe (Lipton), with added ingredients	½ cup	60
Pasta Shells with Sauce (Banquet Gourmet)	10 oz	178
Ravioli, Beef, in Meat Sauce (Franco-American)	7½ oz	20
RavioliOs, Beef, in Meat Sauce (Franco-American)	7½ oz	20

**Contains less than 20 milligrams of calcium.*

Food	*Portion*	*Calcium (mg)*
Romanoff International Noodle Mix (Betty Crocker), with added ingredients	¼ pkg	80
Sour Cream & Chive Noodles & Sauce (Lipton), with added ingredients	½ cup	*
Spaghetti—See Also Prepared Main Dishes		
Spaghetti & Italian Sausage (Hormel)	7 ½ oz	56
Spaghetti 'n Beef (Hormel)	7 ½ oz	44
Spaghetti in Meat Sauce (Franco-American)	7 ½ oz	20
Spaghetti with Meatballs in Tomato Sauce (Franco-American)	7⅜ oz	20
Spaghetti with Meatballs (Stouffer's)	12⅝ oz	150
SpaghettiOs in Tomato & Cheese Sauce (Franco-American)	7 ½ oz	20
SpaghettiOs with Meatballs in Tomato Sauce (Franco-American)	7⅜ oz	20
Stroganoff International Noodle Mix (Betty Crocker), with added ingredients	¼ pkg	60
Stroganoff Noodles & Sauce, Deluxe (Lipton), with added ingredients	½ cup	40
UFO's (Franco-American)	7 ½ oz	20

**Contains less than 20 milligrams of calcium.*

SOUPS, SAUCES, AND GRAVIES

Food	*Portion*	*Calcium (mg)*
SOUPS		
Asparagus, Cream of (Campbell's), prepared	8 oz	20
Asparagus, Cream of, condensed, prepared with milk	1 cup	175
Bean 'n Ham, Chunky Old Fashioned (Campbell's) individual service size	11 oz	100
Bean with Bacon (Campbell's), prepared	8 oz	60
Beef Barley, Soup Starter, Homemade (Beatrice)	1.34 oz	30
Beef, Chunky (Campbell's) 19 oz size	9½ oz	20
Beef Flavor Cup-A-Soup, Lots-A-Noodles (Lipton)	7 fl oz	20
Celery, Cream of, condensed, prepared with milk	1 cup	186
Celery, Cream of, condensed, prepared with water	1 cup	40

Food	*Portion*	*Calcium (mg)*
Soups, *continued*		
Cheddar Cheese (Campbell's), prepared	8 oz	80
Cheese, condensed, prepared with milk	1 cup	288
Cheese, condensed, prepared with water	1 cup	142
Chicken and Dumplings, condensed, prepared with water	1 cup	15
Chicken, Cream of (Campbell's), prepared	8 oz	20
Chicken Gumbo (Campbell's), prepared	8 oz	20
Chicken, Hearty, Country Style Cup-A-Soup (Lipton)	6 fl oz	*
Chicken Mushroom, condensed, prepared with water	1 cup	29
Chicken Noodle with Mushrooms, Chunky (Campbell's) 19 oz size	9½ oz	20
Chicken Vegetable, Chunky, Low Sodium (Campbell's)	10¾ oz	40
Chili Beef, Chunky (Campbell's) 19½ oz size	9¾ oz	60
Clam Chowder, Manhattan (Campbell's), prepared	8 oz	20
Clam Chowder, New England, Chunky (Campbell's) individual service size	10¾ oz	40

Contains less than 20 milligrams of calcium.

Food	*Portion*	*Calcium (mg)*
Soups, *continued*		
Clam Chowder, New England, condensed, prepared with milk	1 cup	187
Clam Chowder, New England, condensed, prepared with water	1 cup	43
Clam Chowder, New England (Stouffer's)	8 oz	80
Corn Chowder, New England, condensed, reconstituted with milk (Snow's)	7½ oz	150
Escarole, ready-to-serve	1 cup	32
Fish Chowder, New England, condensed, reconstituted with milk (Snow's)	7½ oz	150
Gazpacho (Campbell's), prepared	8 oz	20
Gazpacho, ready-to-serve	1 cup	24
Ground Beef Vegetable Soup Starter, Homemade (Beatrice)	1.29 oz	20
Minestrone (Campbell's), prepared	8 oz	20
Mushroom, Cream of (Campbell's), prepared	8 oz	20
Mushroom, Cream of, condensed, prepared with milk	1 cup	178
Mushroom, Cream of, Low Sodium (Campbell's)	10½ oz	60
Onion, condensed, prepared with water	1 cup	26

Food	*Portion*	*Calcium (mg)*
Soups, *continued*		
Onion, Cream of, condensed, prepared with milk	1 cup	180
Onion, Cream of, condensed, prepared with water	1 cup	34
Onion, French (Campbell's), prepared	8 oz	20
Onion, French, Low Sodium (Campbell's)	10½ oz	20
Oriental Style Cup-A-Soup, Lots-A-Noodles (Lipton)	7 fl oz	20
Oyster Stew, condensed, prepared with milk	1 cup	167
Oyster Stew, condensed, prepared with water	1 cup	22
Pea, Green, Cup-A-Soup (Lipton)	6 fl oz	20
Pea, Split, Low Sodium (Campbell's)	10¾ oz	40
Pea, Split, 'n Ham, Chunky (Campbell's) 19 oz size	9½ oz	20
Pea, Split, with Ham (Stouffer's)	8¼ oz	20
Potato, Cream of (Campbell's), prepared	8 oz	*
Potato, Cream of, condensed, prepared with milk	1 cup	166
Potato, Cream of, condensed, prepared with water	1 cup	20

**Contains less than 20 milligrams of calcium.*

Food	Portion	Calcium (mg)
Soups, *continued*		
Seafood Chowder, New England, condensed, reconstituted with milk (Snow's)	7 1/2 oz	150
Sirloin Burger, Chunky (Campbell's) 19 oz size	9 1/2 oz	20
Sirloin Burger, Chunky (Campbell's) individual service size	10 3/4 oz	20
Spinach, Cream of (Stouffer)	8 oz	200
Tomato Bisque (Campbell's), prepared	8 oz	40
Tomato Bisque, condensed, prepared with water	1 cup	40
Tomato (Campbell's), prepared	8 oz	*
Tomato (Campbell's), with 4 oz soup and 4 oz milk	8 oz	150
Tomato, condensed, prepared with milk	1 cup	159
Tomato, Cream of,		
Tomato Cup-A-Soup (Lipton)	6 fl oz	20
Tomato Onion (Lipton)	8 fl oz	20
Tomato Rice, condensed, prepared with water	1 cup	23
Vegetable Beef, Chunky, Low Sodium (Campbell's)	10 3/4 oz	40
Vegetable (Campbell's), prepared	8 oz	20

Contains less than 20 milligrams of calcium.

Food	*Portion*	*Calcium (mg)*
Soups, *continued*		
Vegetable, Chunky (Campbell's) individual service size	10¾ oz	60
Vegetable, Harvest, Country Style Cup-A-Soup (Lipton)	6 fl oz	20
Vegetable with Beef Broth, condensed, prepared with water	1 cup	18
SAUCES		
Barbecue	1 cup	48
Cheese, prepared with milk	1 cup	570
Chili, bottled	1 tbsp.	3
Enchilada, Hot, cooking sauce (Del Monte)	½ cup	20
Enchilada, Mild, cooking sauce (Del Monte)	½ cup	20
Hollandaise (French's), prepared with water	3 tbsp.	20
Hollandaise, with butterfat	1 cup	130
Pizza, with Cheese (Contadina)	¼ cup	26
Pizza, with Tomato Chunks (Contadina)	¼ cup	20
Salsa, Chile, Green, Mild (Del Monte)	¼ cup	20
Salsa, Picante, hot and chunky (Del Monte)	¼ cup	20
Salsa, Picante, hot (Del Monte)	¼ cup	20
Spaghetti	1 serving	17

Food	*Portion*	*Calcium (mg)*
Sauces, *continued*		
Spaghetti, canned	1 cup	70
Spaghetti, No Salt Added (Hunt's)	4 oz	20
Spaghetti, with Mushrooms	1 serving	40
Spaghetti, with Mushrooms (Prego)	4 oz	20
Stroganoff	1 cup	371
Sweet 'n Sour, International (Contadina)	4 oz	28
Sweet and Sour, prepared with water and vinegar	1 cup	41
Tartar	1 tbsp.	3
Teriyaki	1 cup	112
Tomato (Del Monte)	1 cup	20
Tomato Herb (Hunt's)	4 oz	20
Tomato, Italian (Hunt's)	4 oz	20
Tomato, No Salt Added (Del Monte)	1 cup	20
Tomato, with Cheese (Hunt's)	4 oz	60
White, prepared with milk	1 cup	424
GRAVIES		
Beef, canned	1 cup	14
Chicken, canned	1 cup	48
Chicken, dehydrated, prepared with water	1 cup	39
Mushroom, canned	1 cup	17
Mushroom, dehydrated, prepared with water	1 cup	49
Onion, dehydrated, prepared with water	1 cup	69

PREPARED MAIN DISHES

Food	Portion	Calcium (mg)
PREPARED MAIN DISHES		
Beanee Weenee (Van Camp's)	1 cup	95
Beans & Franks—See Also Vegetables		
Beans and Franks (Banquet)	1 dinner	153
Beef and Spinach Stuffed Pasta Shells with Tomato Sauce (Stouffer's)	9 oz	150
Beef Burgundy Dinner Classies (Armour)	1 dinner	40
Beef, Chipped, Creamed, Cookin' Bag Entrees (Banquet)	4 oz	112
Beef, Chipped, Creamed, (Stouffer's)	5 1/2 oz	100
Beef Chop Suey with Rice (Stouffer's)	12 oz	20
Beef, Chopped (Banquet)	1 dinner	69
Beef, Chopped, Extra Helping Dinner (Banquet)	18 oz	104
Beef, Chunky, frozen pie (Swanson)	1 pie	20

Food	*Portion*	*Calcium (mg)*
Prepared Main Dishes, *continued*		
Beef, Extra Helping Dinner (Banquet)	16 oz	97
Beef, frozen dinner (Swanson)	1 dinner	20
Beef, frozen meat pie, Hungry-Man (Swanson)	1 pie	20
Beef, frozen, meat pie (Swanson)	1 pie	20
Beef Pie (Stouffer's)	10 oz	40
Beef Pizza Patties, Entree Express (Banquet)	3 oz	68
Beef Ribs, Boneless, Dinner Classics (Armour)	1 dinner	100
Beef, Sliced, frozen dinner, Hungry-Man (Swanson)	1 dinner	40
Beef, Sliced, frozen entree, Hungry-Man (Swanson)	1 entree	20
Beef Steak, Chopped, frozen dinner, Hungry-Man (Swanson)	1 dinner	60
Beef Stew (Dinty Moore)	7½ oz	19
Beef Stew, Family Entree (Banquet)	8 oz	23
Beef Stew (Stouffer's)	10 oz	20
Beef Stroganoff, Dinner Classics (Armour)	1 dinner	100
Beef Stroganoff, frozen dinner, Le Menu (Swanson)	1 dinner	150
Beef Stroganoff with Parsley Noodles (Stouffer's)	9¾ oz	60

Food	Portion	Calcium (mg)
Prepared Main Dishes, *continued*		
Beef Teriyaki in Sauce with Rice and Vegetables (Stouffer's)	9¾ oz	40
Beef with Gravy (Banquet)	1 dinner	59
Burrito, Bean & Beef, frozen dinner (Swanson)	1 dinner	150
Burrito, Fried, Crispy, frozen (Van de Kamp's)	6 oz	50
Burrito, Grande, with Rice and Corn, frozen (Van de Kamp's)	14¾ oz	200
Burrito, Sirloin, Grande, frozen (Van de Kamp's)	11 oz	200
Cabbage Rolls, Stuffed with Beef, in Tomato Sauce (Green Giant)	7 oz	50
Cheese Souffle (Stouffer's)	6 oz	300
Cheese-Stuffed Pasta Shells with Meat Sauce (Stouffer's)	9 oz	400
Chicken & Dumplings, canned (Swanson)	7½ oz	20
Chicken a la King, canned (Swanson)	5¼ oz	40
Chicken a la King, Cookin' Bag Entrees (Banquet)	5 oz	128
Chicken, Almond Cantonese, with Rice, frozen (Van de Kamp's)	11 oz.	100
Chicken and Broccoli with Rice in Cheese Sauce (Green Giant)	9.5 oz.	200

Food	*Portion*	*Calcium (mg)*
Prepared Main Dishes, *continued*		
Chicken Cacciatore (Green Giant)	9 oz	50
Chicken Cashew in Sauce with Rice (Stouffer's)	9½ oz	20
Chicken, Creamed (Stouffer's)	6½ oz	60
Chicken Crepes with Mushroom Sauce (Stouffer's)	8¼ oz	150
Chicken Divan (Stouffer's)	8½ oz	200
Chicken, Escalloped, and Noodles (Stouffer's)	5¾ oz	40
Chicken Florentine, frozen dinner, Le Menu (Swanson)	1 dinner	150
Chicken Fricassee, Dinner Classics (Armour)	1 dinner	100
Chicken, Fried, Assorted Pieces, frozen (Swanson)	3¼ oz (edible portion)	20
Chicken, Fried, Assorted Pieces, Take-Out, frozen (Swanson)	3¼ oz (edible portion)	20
Chicken, Fried (Banquet)	1 dinner	89
Chicken, Fried, Barbecue Flavor, frozen dinner (Swanson)	1 dinner	40
Chicken, Fried, Breast Portions, frozen dinner (Swanson)	1 dinner	60
Chicken, Fried, Breast Portions, frozen dinner, Hungry-Man (Swanson)	1 dinner	60

Food	*Portion*	*Calcium (mg)*
Prepared Main Dishes, *continued*		
Chicken, Fried, Dark Meat, frozen dinner (Swanson)	1 dinner	60
Chicken, Fried, Dark Portions, frozen dinner, Hungry-Man (Swanson)	1 dinner	60
Chicken, Fried, Dark Portions, frozen entree, Hungry-Man (Swanson)	1 entree	60
Chicken, Fried, frozen entree (Swanson)	1 entree	40
Chicken, frozen meat pie, Hungry-Man (Swanson)	1 pie	60
Chicken, frozen meat pie (Swanson)	1 pie	20
Chicken, Hawaiian, Dinner Classics (Armour)	1 dinner	80
Chicken Milan, Dinner Classics (Armour)	1 dinner	70
Chicken Nibbles, frozen entree (Swanson)	1 entree	20
Chicken Nibbles, wing sections, frozen (Swanson)	3 ¼ oz (edible portion)	20
Chicken Paprikash with Egg Noodles (Stouffer's)	10 ½ oz	60
Chicken Parmigiana, Breast of, frozen dinner, Le Menu (Swanson)	1 dinner	150
Chicken Parmigiana, Family Entree (Banquet)	6.4 oz	83
Chicken Parmigiana, frozen dinner, Hungry-Man (Swanson)	1 dinner	300

Food	Portion	Calcium (mg)
Prepared Main Dishes, *continued*		
Chicken Patties, BBQ, Breaded, Entree Express (Banquet)	3 oz	24
Chicken Patties, Italian Flavored, Entree Express (Banquet)	3 oz	24
Chicken Pie (Stouffer's)	10 oz	80
Chicken Provencale (Green Giant)	10 oz	50
Chicken Stew, canned (Swanson)	7⅝ oz	20
Chicken-Stuffed Pasta Shells with Cheese Sauce (Stouffer's)	9 oz	350
Chicken Suiza with Rice and Beans, frozen (Van de Kamp's)	14¾ oz	450
Chicken, Sweet & Sour, frozen dinner, Le Menu (Swanson)	1 dinner	80
Chicken, Sweet and Sour, Dinner Classics (Armour)	1 dinner	80
Chicken Teriyaki, Dinner Classics (Armour)	1 dinner	60
Chicken Thighs & Drumsticks, frozen (Swanson)	3¼ oz (edible portion)	20
Chilee Weenee (Van Camp's)	1 cup	68
Chili Con Carne with Beans (Stouffer's)	8¾ oz	80
Chili Mac (Hormel)	7½ oz	41
Chili-Mac (Wolf)	scant cup	28
Chili, No Beans (Hormel)	7½ oz	60

Food	*Portion*	*Calcium (mg)*
Prepared Main Dishes, *continued*		
Chili with Beans (Hormel)	7 1/2 oz	78
Chili with Beans, Hot (Hormel)	7 1/2 oz	70
Chili with Beans (Van Camp's)	1 cup	63
Chili with Beans (Wolf)	1 cup	59
Chili without Beans, Extra Spicy (Wolf)	scant cup	60
Chili without Beans (Van Camp's)	1 cup	46
Chili without Beans (Wolf)	1 cup	64
Chow Mein, Beef Mandarin, frozen (Van de Kamp's)	11 oz.	100
Chow Mein, Chicken Mandarin, frozen (Van de Kamp's)	11 oz.	100
Enchilada, Beef and Cheese, with Rice and Beans, frozen (Van de Kamp's)	14 3/4 oz	350
Enchilada, Beef, Dinner, frozen (Van de Kamp's)	12 oz	200
Enchilada, Beef, Family Entree (Banquet)	8 oz	52
Enchilada, Beef, frozen entree, Hungry-Man (Swanson)	1 entree	200
Enchilada, Beef, frozen entree (Swanson)	1 entree	100
Enchilada, Beef, frozen (Van de Kamp's)	7 1/2 oz	150
Enchilada, Beef, International Favorites Dinners (Banquet)	12 oz	109

Food	Portion	Calcium (mg)
Prepared Main Dishes, *continued*		
Enchilada, Cheese, with Rice and Beans, frozen (Van de Kamp's)	14¾ oz	500
Enchilada, Chicken, frozen (Van de Kamp's)	7½ oz	200
Fish 'n' Chips, frozen dinner, Hungry-Man (Swanson)	1 dinner	100
Fish 'n' Chips, frozen dinner (Swanson)	1 dinner	40
Fish 'n' Chips, frozen entree (Swanson)	1 entree	20
Fish (Banquet)	1 dinner	62
Fish, Fillet of, Dinner, frozen (Van de Kamp's)	12 oz	250
Fish Parmesan, frozen (Mrs. Paul's)	5 oz	100
Flounder Fillet with Salmon Mousse, frozen dinner, Le Menu (Swanson)	1 dinner	100
Green Peppers, Stuffed, Dinner Classics (Armour)	1 dinner	80
Green Peppers, Stuffed with Beef, in Tomato Sauce (Green Giant)	7 oz	*
Green Peppers Stuffed with Beef in Tomato Sauce (Stouffer)	7¾ oz	150
Ham and Asparagus Crepes (Stouffer's)	6¼ oz	150

**Contains less than 20 milligrams of calcium.*

Food	*Portion*	*Calcium (mg)*
Prepared Main Dishes, *continued*		
Ham and Swiss Cheese Crepes with Cream Sauce (Stouffer's)	7 1/2 oz	400
Ham Steak, frozen dinner, Le Menu (Swanson)	1 dinner	60
Hamburger Helper, Beef Noodle (Betty Crocker) with 1/5 lb ground beef	1/5 pkg	20
Hamburger Helper, Beef Romanoff (Betty Crocker) with 1/5 lb ground beef	1/5 pkg	60
Hamburger Helper, Cheeseburger Macaroni (Betty Crocker) with 1/5 lb ground beef	1/5 pkg	60
Hamburger Helper, Chili Tomato (Betty Crocker) with 1/5 lb ground beef	1/5 pkg	20
Hamburger Helper, Hamburger Hash (Betty Crocker) with 1/5 lb ground beef	1/5 pkg	20
Hamburger Helper, Hamburger Pizza Dish (Betty Crocker) with 1/5 lb ground beef	1/5 pkg	20
Hamburger Helper, Hamburger Stew (Betty Crocker) with 1/5 lb ground beef	1/5 pkg	20
Hamburger Helper, Lasagne (Betty Crocker) with 1/5 lb ground beef	1/5 pkg	20

Food	Portion	Calcium (mg)
Prepared Main Dishes, *continued*		
Hamburger Helper, Potatoes Au Gratin (Betty Crocker) with ⅕ lb ground beef	⅕ pkg	20
Hamburger Helper, Spaghetti (Betty Crocker) with ⅕ lb ground beef	⅕ pkg	20
Hamburger Mate Burger 'N Cheese Dinner, prepared with meat (Creamette)	⅕ pkg	100
Italian Style International Favorites Dinners (Banquet)	12 oz	79
Lasagna—See Noodles and Pasta		
Macaroni—See Noodles and Pasta		
Meatballs, Swedish, Dinner Classics (Armour)	1 dinner	100
Meatballs, Swedish, in Gravy with Parsley Noodles (Stouffer's)	11 oz	60
Meat Loaf, frozen dinner (Swanson)	1 dinner	100
Meat Loaf with Tomato Sauce, frozen entree (Swanson)	1 entree	60
Mexican frozen dinner, Hungry-Man (Swanson)	1 dinner	350
Mexican-Style Combination, frozen dinner (Swanson)	1 dinner	150

Food	*Portion*	*Calcium (mg)*
Prepared Main Dishes, *continued*		
Mexican-Style Combination International Favorites Dinners (Banquet)	12 oz	194
Mexican-Style Dinner, frozen (Van de Kamp's)	11 ½ oz	150
Mexican-Style Extra Helping Dinner (Banquet)	21.25 oz	411
Mexican Style International Favorites Dinners (Banquet)	12 oz	110
Mostaccioli and Meat Sauce Family Entree (Banquet)	8 oz	30
Noodle Dinners—See Also Noodles and Pasta		
Noodle Weenee (Van Camp's)	1 cup	47
Noodles & Chicken, frozen dinner (Swanson)	1 dinner	40
Omelet, Spanish-Style, frozen breakfast (Swanson)	1 breakfast	80
Omelets with Cheese Sauce & Ham, frozen breakfast (Swanson)	1 breakfast	250
Pancakes & Blueberry Sauce, frozen breakfast (Swanson)	1 breakfast	60
Pancakes & Sausages, frozen breakfast (Swanson)	1 breakfast	80
Pancakes with Strawberries, frozen breakfast (Swanson)	1 breakfast	60

Food	*Portion*	*Calcium (mg)*
Prepared Main Dishes, *continued*		
Pasta Dinners—See Noodles and Pasta		
Pepper Steak, frozen dinner, Le Menu (Swanson)	1 dinner	40
Pizza, Bacon, Canadian-Style, frozen, 7¾ oz (Celeste)	1 pizza	491
Pizza, Bacon, Canadian-Style, frozen, 19 oz (Celeste)	¼ pizza	301
Pizza, Cheese, baked, 4¾-inch sector (⅛ of 12-inch diameter pie)	1 sector	86
Pizza, Cheese, frozen, 6½ oz (Celeste)	1 pizza	375
Pizza, Cheese, frozen, 17¾ oz (Celeste)	¼ pizza	204
Pizza, Deluxe, frozen, 8¼ oz (Celeste)	1 pizza	332
Pizza, Deluxe, frozen, 22¼ oz (Celeste)	¼ pizza	267
Pizza, French Bread, Cheese (Stouffer's)	5 3/16 oz	200
Pizza, French Bread, Deluxe (Stouffer's)	6 3/16 oz	200
Pizza, French Bread, Hamburger (Stouffer's)	6⅛ oz	200
Pizza, French Bread, Pepperoni (Stouffer's)	5⅝ oz	200
Pizza, French Bread, Sausage and Mushroom (Stouffer's)	6¼ oz	100
Pizza, French Bread, Sausage (Stouffer's)	6 oz	200

Food	*Portion*	*Calcium (mg)*
Prepared Main Dishes, *continued*		
Pizza, Pepperoni, frozen, 6¾ oz (Celeste)	1 pizza	336
Pizza, Pepperoni, frozen, 19 oz (Celeste)	¼ pizza	186
Pizza, Sausage and Mushroom, frozen, 8½ oz (Celeste)	1 pizza	362
Pizza, Sausage and Mushroom, frozen, 22½ oz (Celeste)	¼ pizza	310
Pizza, Sausage, frozen, 7½ oz (Celeste)	1 pizza	371
Pizza, Sausage, frozen, 20 oz (Celeste)	¼ pizza	322
Pizza Suprema, frozen, 9 oz (Celeste)	1 pizza	454
Pizza Suprema, frozen, 23 oz (Celeste)	¼ pizza	295
Polynesian-Style frozen dinner (Swanson)	1 dinner	60
Pork and Beans (Hunt's)	4 oz	40
Pork, Loin of, frozen dinner (Swanson)	1 dinner	20
Pork, Sweet and Sour, Dinner Classics (Armour)	1 dinner	100
Pork, Sweet and Sour, with Rice, frozen (Van de Kamp's)	11 oz	50
Pot Roast, Yankee, Dinner Classics (Armour)	1 dinner	50
Pot Roast, Yankee, frozen dinner, Le Menu (Swanson)	1 dinner	40

Food	Portion	Calcium (mg)
Prepared Main Dishes, *continued*		
Ravioli—See Noodles and Pasta		
Rice, Spanish—See Rice		
Roast Beef Hash (Mary Kitchen)	7½ oz	52
Salisbury Steak (Banquet)	1 dinner	62
Salisbury Steak, Dinner Classics (Armour)	1 dinner	80
Salisbury Steak, Extra Helping Dinner (Banquet)	19 oz	127
Salisbury Steak, frozen dinner, Hungry-Man (Swanson)	1 dinner	200
Salisbury Steak, frozen dinner (Swanson)	1 dinner	80
Salisbury Steak, frozen entree, Hungry-Man (Swanson)	1 entree	100
Salisbury Steak, frozen entree (Swanson)	1 entree	40
Salisbury Steak, frozen main course entree (Swanson)	1 entree	40
Salisbury Steaks, with Onion Gravy (Stouffer's)	6 oz	20
Scallops and Shrimp Mariner with Rice (Stouffer's)	10¼ oz	150
Seafood Newburg, Dinner Classics (Armour)	1 dinner	200
Shells and Cheese Dinner (Velveeta)	¾ cup	200
Shrimp Creole with Rice (Green Giant)	9 oz	50

Food	*Portion*	*Calcium (mg)*
LOW-CALORIE PREPARED MAIN DISHES		
Beef and Pork Cannelloni with Mornay Sauce (Lean Cuisine)	9⅝ oz	200
Beef Julienne, Light and Elegant Entrees (Banquet)	8.5 oz.	27
Beef, Oriental, with Vegetables and Rice (Lean Cuisine)	8⅝ oz	20
Beef Pepper Steak (Classic Lites/Armour)	1 dinner	40
Beef, Sliced, and Broccoli (Classic Lites/Armour)	1 dinner	40
Beef Stroganoff (Light and Elegant Entrees/ Banquet)	9 oz	45
Beef Teriyaki (Light and Elegant Entrees/ Banquet)	8 oz	30
Cabbage, Stuffed with Meat, in Tomato Sauce (Lean Cuisine)	10¾ oz	60
Cheese Cannelloni with Tomato Sauce (Lean Cuisine)	9⅛ oz	300
Chicken a l'Orange with Almond Rice (Lean Cuisine)	8 oz	20
Chicken and Vegetables with Vermicelli (Lean Cuisine)	12¾ oz	100

Food	Portion	Calcium (mg)
Low-Calorie Prepared Main Dishes, *continued*		
Chicken, BBQ (Light and Elegant Entrees/ Banquet)	8 oz	22
Chicken Breast Marsala, Medallions of (Classic Lites/Armour)	1 dinner	60
Chicken Burgundy (Classic Lites/Armour)	1 dinner	80
Chicken Cacciatore with Vermicelli (Lean Cuisine)	10⅞ oz	40
Chicken Chow Mein with Rice (Lean Cuisine)	11¼ oz	20
Chicken, Glazed, with Vegetable Rice (Lean Cuisine)	8½ oz	20
Chicken Oriental (Classic Lites/Armour)	1 dinner	40
Chicken Parmigiana (Light and Elegant Entrees/ Banquet)	8 oz	78
Chicken, Sweet and Sour (Classic Lites/Armour)	1 dinner	40
Chicken with Broccoli (Light and Elegant Entrees/Banquet)	9.5 oz.	204
Cod, Filet of, Divan (Classic Lites/Armour)	1 dinner	100
Fish Dijon (Light Seafood Entree/Mrs. Paul's)	8½ oz	80
Fish, Filet of, Divan (Lean Cuisine)	12⅜ oz	200
Fish, Filet of, Florentine (Lean Cuisine)	9 oz	150

Food	Portion	Calcium (mg)
Low-Calorie Prepared Main Dishes, *continued*		
Fish, Filet of, Jardiniere with Souffleed Potatoes (Lean Cuisine)	11 1/4 oz	150
Fish Florentine (Light Seafood Entree/Mrs. Paul's)	9 oz	250
Fish Mornay (Light Seafood Entree/Mrs. Paul's)	10 oz	150
Linguini with Clam Sauce (Lean Cuisine)	9 5/8 oz	20
Macaroni and Cheese (Light and Elegant Entrees/Banquet)	9 oz	238
Meatball Stew (Lean Cuisine)	10 oz	40
Scallops Mediterranean (Light Seafood Entree/ Mrs. Paul's)	11 oz	60
Scallops, Oriental, and Vegetables with Rice (Lean Cuisine)	11 oz	60
Seafood Natural Herbs (Classic Lites/Armour)	1 dinner	100
Seafood Newburg (Light Seafood Entree/Mrs. Paul's)	8 1/2 oz	80
Shrimp, Baby, in Sherried Cream Sauce (Classic Lites/Armour)	1 dinner	150
Shrimp Creole (Light and Elegant Entrees/ Banquet)	10 oz	54

Food	Portion	Calcium (mg)
Low-Calorie Prepared Main Dishes, *continued*		
Shrimp Oriental (Light Seafood Entree/Mrs. Paul's)	11 oz	80
Shrimp Primavera (Light Seafood Entree/Mrs. Paul's)	11 oz	80
Spaghetti and Meat Sauce (Light and Elegant Entrees/Banquet)	10.25 oz	100
Spaghetti with Beef and Mushroom Sauce (Lean Cuisine)	11 ½ oz	60
Spaghetti—See Also Noodles and Pasta		
Steak Diane (Classic Lites/ Armour)	1 dinner	80
Steak, Salisbury, with Italian Style Sauce and Vegetables (Lean Cuisine)	9 ½ oz	150
Turf and Surf (Classic Lites/Armour)	1 dinner	60
Turkey Parmesan (Classic Lites/Armour)	1 dinner	150
Veal Pepper Steak (Classic Lites/Armour)	1 dinner	80

CONDIMENTS

Food	*Portion*	*Calcium (mg)*
Allspice, ground	1 tbsp	40
Basil, ground	1 tbsp	95
Basil Leaves, ground (McCormick)	1 tsp	23
Beef Stew seasoning mix (French's), package contents only	1/6 pkg	20
Caramel Topping, Chocolate (Kraft)	1 tbsp	20
Caramel Topping (Kraft)	1 tbsp	20
Caraway Seed	1 tbsp	46
Catsup, Tomato (bottled)	1 tbsp	3
Celery Seed	1 tbsp	115
Celery Seed, ground (McCormick)	1 tsp	43
Chili Powder	1 tbsp	21
Chocolate Topping (Kraft)	1 tbsp	20
Cinnamon, ground	1 tbsp	84
Cinnamon, ground (McCormick)	1 tsp	27
Cloves, ground	1 tbsp	43
Coriander Seed	1 tbsp	35
Cumin Seed	1 tbsp	56
Curry Powder	1 tbsp	30

Food	*Portion*	*Calcium (mg)*
Dill Seed	1 tbsp	100
Dill Seed, ground (McCormick)	1 tsp	34
Dressing, Salad, Blue Cheese	1 cup	199
Dressing, Salad, French, low calorie	1 cup	29
Dressing, Salad, French, regular	1 cup	28
Dressing, Salad, Italian, regular	1 cup	23
Dressing, Salad, Russian	1 cup	47
Dressing, Salad, Thousand Island	1 cup	28
Dressing, Salad (Wish-Bone), all flavors	1 tbsp	*
Dressing, Salad (Wish-Bone Lite), all flavors	1 tbsp	*
Dressing, Sour, made with nonfat dry milk	1 cup	300
Dressing, Sour, made with nonfat dry milk	1 tbsp	20
Fennel Seed	1 tbsp	69
Fennel Seed, ground (McCormick)	1 tsp	27
Jams and Preserves	1 tbsp	4
Marjoram, dried	1 tbsp	34
Marjoram, ground (McCormick)	1 tsp	30
Mayonnaise	1 cup	40
Molasses, Blackstrap	1 tbsp	137
Mustard, Brown, prepared	1 cup	310
Mustard, Brown, prepared	1 tsp	6
Mustard, Dijon (French's)	1 tbsp	*

**Contains less than 20 milligrams of calcium.*

Food	*Portion*	*Calcium (mg)*
Mustard, Yellow, prepared	1 cup	210
Mustard, Yellow, prepared	1 tsp	4
Mustard, Yellow, prepared (French's)	1 tbsp	*
Oregano, ground	1 tbsp	71
Oregano, ground (McCormick)	1 tsp	27
Parsley, dried	1 tbsp	19
Pepper, Black	1 tbsp	28
Poppy Seed	1 tbsp	127
Poppy Seed, ground (McCormick)	1 tsp	40
Poultry Seasoning	1 tbsp	37
Sage, ground	1 tbsp	33
Savory, ground (McCormick)	1 tsp	31
Seasonings, Taco, Meat, Mild (Ortega)	1 oz	41
Sesame Tahini (Sahadi)	2 tbsp	20
Syrup, fudge type	1 fl oz or 2 tbsp	48
Thyme, ground	1 tbsp	81
Thyme, ground (McCormick)	1 tsp	31

*Contains less than 20 milligrams of calcium.

DESSERTS

Food	*Portion*	*Calcium (mg)*
CAKE		
Angel Food (1/16 of 9¾ inch diameter tube cake)	1 piece	40
Apple (Duncan Hines Deluxe Cake Mix), with added ingredients	1/12 cake	60
Applesauce Raisin Snackin' Cake Mix (Betty Crocker)	1/9 pkg	40
Applesauce Spice Cake Mix (Pillsbury Plus), with added ingredients	1/12 cake	40
Banana Cake Mix (Pillsbury Plus), with added ingredients	1/12 cake	40
Banana Supermoist Cake Mix (Betty Crocker), with added ingredients	1/12 pkg	60
Banana Supreme (Duncan Hines Deluxe Cake Mix), with added ingredients	1/12 cake	60
Banana Walnut Snackin' Cake Mix (Betty Crocker)	1/9 pkg	40
Black Forest Cake (Sara Lee)	1/8 cake	20

Food	Portion	Calcium (mg)
Cakes, *continued*		
Boston Cream, Classics Dessert Mix (Betty Crocker), with added ingredients	1/8 pkg	150
Boston Cream Pie (Mrs. Smith's)	1/8 cake	26
Boston Cream Pie (1/12 of 8 inch diameter cake)	1 piece	40
Boston Cream Supreme (Pepperidge Farm)	2 7/8 oz.	20
Brownie Fudge Mix (Pillsbury), with added ingredients	one 2-inch square	*
Butter Pecan Supermoist Cake Mix (Betty Crocker), with added ingredients	1/12 pkg	40
Butter Recipe Cake Mix (Pillsbury Plus), with added ingredients	1/12 cake	40
Butter Recipe Yellow Supermoist Cake Mix (Betty Crocker), with added ingredients	1/12 pkg	60
Butterscotch Pecan Layer (Pepperidge Farm)	1 5/8 oz	20
Caramel with Caramel Icing (2-layer cake)	1/12 cake	60
Carrot 'n Spice Cake Mix (Pillsbury Plus), with added ingredients	1/12 cake	40
Carrot (Duncan Hines Deluxe Cake Mix), with added ingredients	1/12 cake	60

Contains less than 20 milligrams of calcium.

Food	Portion	Calcium (mg)
Cakes, *continued*		
Cheese Cake, Chocolate Chip, Elegant Endings (Sara Lee)	1/6 cake	60
Cheese Cake, Classic Elegant Endings (Sara Lee)	1/6 cake	60
Cheese Cake, Cream French (Sara Lee)	1/8 cake	40
Cheese Cake, Cream French Strawberry (Sara Lee)	1/8 cake	20
Cheese Cake, Pecan Praline, Elegant Endings (Sara Lee)	1/6 cake	60
Cheese Cake, Real, No-Bake Mix, prepared (Royal)	1/8 pie	150
Cheese Cake, Real, No-Bake Mix (Royal)	1 3/8 oz	80
Cherry Chip Supermoist Cake Mix (Betty Crocker), with added ingredients	1/12 pkg	*
Cherry Supreme (Duncan Hines Deluxe Cake Mix), with added ingredients	1/12 cake	60
Chocolate Chip (Duncan Hines Deluxe Cake Mix), with added ingredients	1/12 cake	60
Chocolate Chip Golden Snackin' Cake Mix (Betty Crocker)	1/9 pkg	60

Contains less than 20 milligrams of calcium.

Food	*Portion*	*Calcium (mg)*
Cakes, *continued*		
Chocolate Chocolate Chip Supermoist Cake Mix (Betty Crocker), with added ingredients	1/12 pkg	60
Chocolate, Deep (Duncan Hines Deluxe Cake Mix), with added ingredients	1/12 cake	60
Chocolate, Dutch, Supreme (Pepperidge Farm)	1 3/4 oz.	20
Chocolate Fudge Chip Snackin' Cake Mix (Betty Crocker)	1/9 pkg	60
Chocolate Mint Layer (Pepperidge Farm)	1 5/8 oz	20
Chocolate Mousse Bundt Ring Cake Mix (Pillsbury), with added ingredients	1/16 cake	40
Chocolate Pudding Classics Dessert Mix (Betty Crocker), with added ingredients	1/6 pkg	40
Chocolate Sour Cream (Duncan Hines Deluxe Cake Mix), with added ingredients	1/12 cake	60
Chocolate Supreme (Pepperidge Farm)	2 7/8 oz	20
Chocolate, Swiss (Duncan Hines Deluxe Cake Mix), with added ingredients	1/12 cake	100

Food	Portion	Calcium (mg)
Cakes, *continued*		
Cinnamon Streusel Swirl Cake Mix (Pillsbury Plus), with added ingredients	1/16 cake	40
Coconut Pecan Snackin' Cake Mix (Betty Crocker)	1/9 pkg	60
Coffee Cake Easy Mix (Aunt Jemima), with added ingredients	1/8 coffee cake	60
Crumb Cakes (Hostess)	1 each	20
Cupcake, Chocolate (Hostess)	1 each	20
Cupcake, Devil's Food, chocolate filling and chocolate frosting (Pillsbury Plus), with added ingredients	1 cupcake	20
Cupcake, Devil's Food, vanilla filling and chocolate frosting (Pillsbury), with added ingredients	1 cupcake	20
Cupcake, Orange (Hostess)	1 each	20
Cupcake, Yellow, vanilla filling and chocolate frosting (Pillsbury), with added ingredients	1 cupcake	40
Dark Chocolate Cake Mix (Pillsbury Plus), with added ingredients	1/12 cake	100
Date Nut Roll (Dromedary)	1/2 inch slice	20
Dessert Cups (Hostess)	1 each	20

Food	Portion	Calcium (mg)
Cakes, *continued*		
Devil's Food Cake Mix (Pillsbury Plus), with added ingredients	1/12 cake	100
Devil's Food (Duncan Hines Deluxe Cake Mix), with added ingredients	1/12 cake	60
Devil's Food, made with eggs and water, with chocolate icing (2-layer cake)	1 piece	40
Dutch Apple Streusel Swirl Cake Mix (Pillsbury), with added ingredients	1/16 cake	20
Fruit Cake, dark, made with enriched flour (1/30 of 1 lb loaf)	1 slice	20
Fudge (Duncan Hines Deluxe Cake Mix), with added ingredients	1/12 cake	20
Fudge Marble Cake Mix (Pillsbury Plus), with added ingredients	1/12 cake	40
Fudge Marble (Duncan Hines Deluxe Cake Mix), with added ingredients	1/12 cake	60
Fudge Marble Streusel Swirl Cake Mix (Pillsbury), with added ingredients	1/16 cake	20
Fudge Peanut Butter Chip Snackin' Cake Mix (Betty Crocker)	1/9 pkg.	60

Food	*Portion*	*Calcium (mg)*
Cakes, *continued*		
Fudge, Tunnel of, Bundt Ring Cake Mix (Pillsbury), with added ingredients	1/16 cake	20
German Black Forest Classics Dessert Mix (Betty Crocker), with added ingredients	1/12 pkg	60
German Chocolate Cake Mix (Pillsbury Plus), with added ingredients	1/12 cake	40
German Chocolate Coconut Pecan Snackin' Cake Mix (Betty Crocker)	1/9 pkg	60
German Chocolate Mix, Stir 'n Streusel (Betty Crocker)	1/6 pkg	20
German Chocolate Supermoist Cake Mix (Betty Crocker), with added ingredients	1/12 pkg	60
Gingerbread Mix (Pillsbury), with added ingredients	one 3 inch square	40
Ho Hos (Hostess)	1 each	20
Lemon Cake Mix (Pillsbury Plus), with added ingredients	1/12 cake	40
Lemon Pudding Classics Dessert Mix (Betty Crocker), with added ingredients	1/6 pkg	40

Food	Portion	Calcium (mg)
Cakes, *continued*		
Lemon Streusel Swirl Cake Mix (Pillsbury), with added ingredients	1/16 cake	60
Lemon Supermoist Cake Mix (Betty Crocker), with added ingredients	1/12 pkg	*
Marble Supermoist Cake Mix (Betty Crocker), with added ingredients	1/12 pkg	40
Milk Chocolate Supermoist Cake Mix (Betty Crocker), with added ingredients	1/12 pkg	40
Mint Fudge Chip Snackin' Cake Mix (Betty Crocker)	1/9 pkg	60
Mocha Cake Mix (Pillsbury Plus), with added ingredients	1/12 cake	100
Mousse, Chocolate Bavarian (Sara Lee)	1/8 cake	20
Pineapple Supreme (Duncan Hines Deluxe Cake Mix), with added ingredients	1/12 cake	60
Pineapple Upside-Down Classics Dessert Mix (Betty Crocker), with added ingredients	1/9 pkg	40
Pound Cake Mix, prepared (Dromedary)	1/2 inch slice	20
Pound Cake, Raisin Walnut (Sara Lee)	1/10 cake	20

**Contains less than 20 milligrams of calcium.*

Food	Portion	Calcium (mg)
Cakes, ***continued***		
Shortcake, Strawberry (Sara Lee)	1/8 cake	20
Sno Balls (Hostess)	1 each	20
Sour Cream Chocolate Supermoist Cake Mix (Betty Crocker), with added ingredients	1/12 pkg	60
Sour Cream White Supermoist Cake Mix (Betty Crocker), with added ingredients	1/12 pkg	*
Spice (Duncan Hines Deluxe Cake Mix), with added ingredients	1/12 cake	60
Spice Supermoist Cake Mix (Betty Crocker), with added ingredients	1/12 pkg	60
Sponge tube cake (1/12 of 9 3/4 inch diameter cake)	1 piece	20
Strawberry Cake Mix (Pillsbury Plus), with added ingredients	1/12 cake	40
Strawberry Cream Supreme (Pepperidge Farm)	2 oz	20
Strawberry Supermoist Cake Mix (Betty Crocker), with added ingredients	1/12 pkg	40
Strawberry Supreme (Duncan Hines Deluxe Cake Mix), with added ingredients	1/12 cake	60
Suzy Q's, Banana (Hostess)	1 each	40

**Contains less than 20 milligrams of calcium.*

Food	*Portion*	*Calcium (mg)*
Cakes, *continued*		
Suzy Q's, Chocolate (Hostess)	1 each	20
Tiger Tail (Hostess)	1 each	20
Twinkies (Hostess)	1 each	20
Vanilla, Golden (Duncan Hines Deluxe Cake Mix), with added ingredients	1/12 cake	60
White Cake Mix (Pillsbury Plus), with added ingredients	1/12 cake	20
White (Duncan Hines Deluxe Cake Mix), with added ingredients	1/12 cake	60
White, made with egg whites and water, with chocolate icing (2-layer cake)	1/16 cake	60
White Supermoist Cake Mix (Betty Crocker), with added ingredients	1/12 pkg	60
Yellow Cake Mix (Pillsbury Plus), with added ingredients	1/12 cake	40
Yellow (Duncan Hines Deluxe Cake Mix), with added ingredients	1/12 cake	60
Yellow, made with eggs and water, with chocolate icing (2-layer cake)	1/16 cake	60
Yellow Supermoist Cake Mix (Betty Crocker), with added ingredients	1/12 pkg	60

Food	*Portion*	*Calcium (mg)*
COOKIES		
Almond Supreme Special Collection (Pepperidge Farm)	2 cookies	20
Biscuit, National, Arrowroot (Nabisco)	1 oz	20
Chocolate Chip, Double (Duncan Hines Cookie Mix), with added ingredients	2 cookies	*
Chocolate Chip (Duncan Hines Cookie Mix), with added ingredients	2 cookies	*
Chocolate Chip, Mocha, Old Fashioned (Pepperidge Farm)	3 cookies	20
Chocolate, Milk, Macadamia Special Collection (Pepperidge Farm)	2 cookies	20
Danish, Imported (Nabisco)	1 oz	20
Fig Newtons (Nabisco)	1 oz	20
Fudge Caramel and Peanut Bars, Heyday (Nabisco)	1 oz	60
Fudge Chocolate Chip Raisin, Almost Home (Nabisco)	1 oz	20
Fudge 'n Chocolate Creme Sandwiches, Almost Home (Nabisco)	1 1/8 oz	20
Fudge 'n Vanilla Creme Sandwiches, Almost Home (Nabisco)	1 1/8 oz	20

*Contains less than 20 milligrams of calcium.

Food	Portion	Calcium (mg)
Cookies, *continued*		
Gingersnaps (2 inch diameter)	4 cookies	20
Gingersnaps, Old Fashion (Nabisco)	1 oz	20
Graham, Bugs Bunny (Nabisco)	1 oz	20
Ladyfingers, whole	4 cookies	20
Macaroon, Coconut, Classics Dessert Mix (Betty Crocker)	1/24 pkg	20
Molasses Crisps, Old Fashioned (Pepperidge Farm)	3 cookies	20
Molasses, Pantry (Nabisco)	1 oz	20
Molasses (3 5/8 inch diameter)	1 cookie	20
Oatmeal Creme Sandwiches, Almost Home (Nabisco)	1 1/8 oz	20
Oatmeal Raisin (Duncan Hines Cookie Mix), with added ingredients	2 cookies	20
Peanut Butter, Almost Home (Nabisco)	1 oz	20
Peanut Butter Chocolate Chip, Old Fashioned (Pepperidge Farm)	3 cookies	80
Peanut Butter Creme Sandwiches, Almost Home (Nabisco)	1 1/8 oz	20
Peanut Butter (Duncan Hines Cookie Mix), with added ingredients	2 cookies	*

**Contains less than 20 milligrams of calcium.*

Food	*Portion*	*Calcium (mg)*
Cookies, *continued*		
Peanut Butter Fudge, Almost Home (Nabisco)	1 oz	20
Raisin Applesauce, Iced, Almost Home (Nabisco)	1 oz.	20
Sugar, Golden (Duncan Hines Cookie Mix), with added ingredients	2 cookies	*
CUSTARDS AND PUDDINGS		
Almond Butter Toasted Pudding, instant, prepared (Royal)	1/2 cup	150
Banana Cream Pudding and Pie Filling, cooked, prepared (Royal)	1/2 cup	150
Banana Cream Pudding, instant, prepared (Royal)	1/2 cup	150
Banana Pudding, Snack Pack (Hunt's)	5 oz	40
Banana Pudding Cup (Del Monte)	5 oz	100
Butterscotch Pudding and Pie Filling, cooked, prepared (Royal)	1/2 cup	150
Chocolate Chocolate Chip Pudding, instant, prepared (Royal)	1/2 cup	150
Chocolate Fudge Pudding and Pie Filling, instant, as prepared, (Jell-O)	1/2 cup	150
Chocolate Mint Pudding, instant, prepared (Royal)	1/2 cup	150
Chocolate Pudding and Pie Filling, instant, as prepared (Jell-O)	1/2 cup	150

Contains less than 20 milligrams of calcium.

Food	Portion	Calcium (mg)
Custards and Puddings, *continued*		
Chocolate Pudding and Pie Filling, as prepared (Royal)	1/2 cup	150
Chocolate Pudding, Snack Pack (Hunt's)	5 oz	40
Chocolate Pudding, (Swiss Miss)	4 oz	100
Chocolate Pudding Cup (Del Monte)	5 oz	100
Chocolate Pudding, Double Rich (Swiss Miss)	4 oz	80
Corn Pudding	1 cup	150
Custard, baked, made with milk	1 cup	300
Custard, Egg (Swiss Miss)	4 oz	100
Custard Pudding and Pie Filling, cooked, prepared (Royal)	1/2 cup	150
Dark 'n Sweet Pudding and Pie Filling, cooked, prepared (Royal)	1/2 cup	150
Dark 'n Sweet Pudding, instant, prepared (Royal)	1/2 cup	150
Flan with Caramel Sauce Pudding and Pie Filling, cooked, prepared (Royal)	1/2 cup	150
Lemon Pudding and Pie Filling, instant, prepared, (Jell-O)	1/2 cup	150
Lemon Pudding, instant, prepared (Royal)	1/2 cup	150
Pistachio Nut Pudding, instant, prepared (Royal)	1/2 cup	150

Food	*Portion*	*Calcium (mg)*
Custards and Puddings, *continued*		
Rice Pudding, Snack Pack (Hunt's)	5 oz	60
Rice Pudding, with Raisins	1 cup	250
Tapioca Pudding Cup (Del Monte)	5 oz	100
Tapioca Pudding, Snack Pack (Hunt's)	5 oz	60
Vanilla Pudding (Swiss Miss)	4 oz	100
Vanilla, as prepared, Pudding and Pie Filling (Royal)	1/2 cup	150
Vanilla, instant, as prepared, Pudding and Pie Filling (Jell-O)	1/2 cup	150
Vanilla Pudding, cooked, prepared (Royal)	1/2 cup	150
Vanilla Pudding, instant, prepared (Royal)	1/2 cup	150
Vanilla Pudding, sugar-free, instant, prepared (Royal)	1/2 cup	150
Vanilla Tapioca Pudding, cooked, prepared (Royal)	1/2 cup	150
FROZEN DAIRY DESSERTS AND TOPPINGS		
Dairy Dessert, Lowfat Strawberry, Wild (Baskin-Robbins)	4 oz scoop	175
Ice cream bar, Chip Crunch (Good Humor)	1 bar	60
Ice cream bar, Chocolate Eclair (Good Humor)	1 bar	40
Ice cream bar, Chocolate Fudge Cake (Good Humor)	1 bar	60

Food	Portion	Calcium (mg)
Frozen Dairy Desserts and Toppings, *continued*		
Ice cream bar, Chocolate Malt (Good Humor)	1 bar	60
Ice cream bar, Toasted Almond (Good Humor)	1 bar	40
Ice cream bar, Toasted Caramel (Good Humor)	1 bar	60
Ice cream bar, Vanilla (Good Humor)	1 bar	60
Ice cream bar, Whammys, assorted (Good Humor)	1 bar	20
Ice Cream Bar, Cookies 'n Cream on a Stick (Oreo)	1 bar	60
Ice Cream, Buttered Pecan (Lady Borden)	1/2 cup	80
Ice Cream, Chocolate (Baskin-Robbins)	4 oz scoop	115
Ice Cream, Chocolate Cookies 'n Cream (Oreo)	3 fl oz	60
Ice Cream, Chocolate, Dutch Almond, All Natural (Borden)	1/2 cup	100
Ice Cream, Chocolate, Dutch (Borden)	1/2 cup	80
Ice Cream, Chocolate (Lady Borden)	1/2 cup	80
Ice Cream, Chocolate Mousse Royale (Baskin-Robbins)	4 oz scoop	112
Ice Cream Cookie Sandwich, all flavors, with 2.7 fl oz ice cream (Good Humor)	1 each	60

Food	*Portion*	*Calcium (mg)*
Frozen Dairy Desserts and Toppings, *continued*		
Ice Cream Cookie Sandwich, all flavors, with 4 fl oz ice cream (Good Humor)	1 each	80
Ice Cream, Mint, Cookies 'n Cream (Oreo)	3 fl oz	60
Ice Cream, Pralines 'N Cream (Baskin-Robbins)	4 oz scoop	99
Ice Cream, Rocky Road (Baskin-Robbins)	4 oz scoop	94
Ice Cream Sandwich, Vanilla (Good Humor)	1 each	60
Ice Cream Sandwiches, Cookies 'n Cream (Oreo)	1 sandwich	80
Ice Cream Slice, Cal-Control, Vanilla (Good Humor)	1 slice	60
Ice Cream Slice, Vanilla (Good Humor)	1 slice	60
Ice Cream, Strawberry (Baskin-Robbins)	4 oz scoop	101
Ice Cream, Strawberry (Borden)	½ cup	60
Ice Cream, Vanilla	1 cup	176
Ice Cream, Vanilla, All Natural (Borden)	½ cup	100
Ice Cream, Vanilla (Baskin-Robbins)	4 oz scoop	136
Ice Cream, Vanilla, Cookies 'n Cream (Oreo)	3 fl oz	60
Ice Cream, Vanilla Flavored, artificial flavor added (Borden)	½ cup	80
Ice Cream, Vanilla, French, All Natural (Borden)	½ cup	100

Food	*Portion*	*Calcium (mg)*
Frozen Dairy Desserts and Toppings, *continued*		
Ice Cream, Vanilla, French (Baskin-Robbins)	4 oz scoop	127
Ice Cream, Vanilla, French (Lady Borden)	½ cup	100
Ice Cream, Vanilla, French, soft serve	1 cup	236
Ice Cream, Vanilla (Land O'Lakes)	4 fl oz	80
Ice Milk, Chocolate, All Natural (Borden)	½ cup	100
Ice Milk, Strawberry, All Natural (Borden)	½ cup	100
Ice Milk, Vanilla, All Natural (Borden)	½ cup	100
Sherbet, Lemon (Borden)	½ cup	40
Sherbet, Orange	1 cup	103
Sherbet, Orange (Baskin-Robbins)	4 oz scoop	35
Sherbet, Orange (Borden)	½ cup	40
Topping, Dessert, nondairy, frozen	1 cup	5
Topping, Dessert, nondairy, powdered	1½ oz	7
Topping, Dessert, nondairy, powdered, prepared with whole milk	1 cup	72
Topping, Dessert, nondairy, pressurized	1 cup	4
Topping, Whipped Cream—See Cream, Topping, Whipped		
PIES		
Apple (Hostess)	1 pie	20
Apple Lattice Pie (Mrs. Smith's)	⅛ pie	14

Food	*Portion*	*Calcium (mg)*
Pies, *continued*		
Apple Pie (Mrs. Smith's)	1/8 pie	15
Banana Cream Pie (Banquet)	1/6 pie	32
Banana Cream Pie (Mrs. Smith's)	1/8 pie	39
Berry (Hostess)	1 pie	40
Blackberry Family Size Fruit Pie (Banquet)	1/6 pie	23
Blueberry (Hostess)	1 pie	20
Blueberry Pie (Mrs. Smith's)	1/8 pie	12
Boston Cream Pie—See Cakes		
Cherry (Hostess)	1 pie	20
Cherry Lattice Pie (Mrs. Smith's)	1/8 pie	12
Cherry Pie (Mrs. Smith's)	1/8 pie	34
Chocolate Cream Pie (Banquet)	1/6 pie	38
Chocolate Cream Pie (Mrs. Smith's)	1/8 pie	23
Coconut Custard Pie (Mrs. Smith's)	1/8 pie	123
Egg Custard Pie (Mrs. Smith's)	1/8 pie	156
Lemon Cream Pie (Banquet)	1/6 pie	30
Lemon Cream Pie, naturally flavored (Mrs. Smith's)	1/8 pie	16
Lemon (Hostess)	1 pie	20
Lemon Meringue Pie (Mrs. Smith's)	1/8 pie	15
Natural Juice Apple Pie (Mrs. Smith's)	1/7 pie	13

Food	*Portion*	*Calcium (mg)*
Pies, *continued*		
Old Fashioned Apple Pie (Mrs. Smith's)	1/8 pie	10
Peach Pie (Hostess)	1 pie	40
Peach Pie (Mrs. Smith's)	1/8 pie	13
Pecan Pie (Mrs. Smith's)	1/8 pie	15
Pie Crust Mix, with added ingredients, Flako, (Aunt Jemima)	1/6 9-inch pie crust	40
Pie Shell (Mrs. Smith's)	1/8 shell	3
Pumpkin Custard Pie (Mrs. Smith's)	1/8 pie	97
Pumpkin Family Size Fruit Pie (Banquet)	1/6 pie	53
Strawberry Cream Pie (Banquet)	1/6 pie	30
Strawberry (Hostess)	1 pie	20

CANDIES, SNACKS, AND NUTS

Food	*Portion*	*Calcium (mg)*
CANDIES		
Almond Bar (Cadbury)	2 oz	140
Almond Joy (Peter Paul)	1.55 oz	20
Brazil Nut Bar (Cadbury)	2 oz	140
Caramel Milk Tidbits, Sugar Babies (Nabisco)	1 5/8 oz	20
Caramello Bar (Cadbury)	2 oz	100
Carmel Nip (Pearson's)	1 oz	20
Chocolate Parfait (Pearson's)	1 oz	20
Coffee Nip (Pearson's)	1 oz	20
Coffioca Parfait (Pearson's)	1 oz	20
Dairy Milk Bar (Cadbury)	2 oz	140
Fruit and Nut Bar (Cadbury)	2 oz	120
Good Stuff Bar (Pearson's)	1.79 oz	60
Halvah (Sahadi)	1 oz	20
Hazelnut Bar (Cadbury)	2 oz	140
Kisses, Chocolate (Hershey's)	8 pieces	80
Kit Kat Wafer Bar (Hershey's)	1.5 oz	80
Krisp with Honey (Cadbury)	2 oz	120
Licorice Nip (Pearson's)	1 oz	20

Food	Portion	Calcium (mg)
Prepared Main Dishes, *continued*		
Sirloin Beef, Chopped, frozen dinner (Swanson)	1 dinner	80
Sirloin Tips, Dinner Classics (Armour)	1 dinner	100
Skettee Weenee (Van Camp's)	1 cup	44
Spaghetti & Meatballs, frozen dinner (Swanson)	1 dinner	100
Spaghetti Dinner, American Style (Kraft)	1 cup	60
Spaghetti Dinner, Tangy Italian-Style (Kraft)	1 cup	80
Spaghetti in Tomato Sauce with Breaded Veal, frozen entree (Swanson)	1 entree	40
Spaghetti with Meatballs, Dinner Classics (Armour)	1 dinner	115
Spaghetti with Meat Sauce (Banquet)	1 dinner	29
Spaghetti with Meat Sauce Dinner (Kraft)	1 cup	100
Spaghetti—See Also Noodles and Pasta		
Spinach Crepes with Cheddar Cheese Sauce (Stouffer's)	9½ oz	300
Steak and Green Peppers in Sauce with Rice and Vegetables (Green Giant)	9 oz	*
Steak Burger, frozen meat pie, Hungry-Man (Swanson)	1 pie	40

**Contains less than 20 milligrams of calcium.*

Food	Portion	Calcium (mg)
Prepared Main Dishes, *continued*		
Steak, Green Pepper, with Rice (Stouffer's)	10½ oz	20
Steak Teriyaki, Dinner Classics (Armour)	1 dinner	40
Stew, Brunswick (Dinty Moore)	7½ oz	63
Swiss Steak, frozen dinner (Swanson)	1 dinner	40
Tamales, Beef (Hormel)	7½ oz	22
Tamales with Sauce (Van Camp's)	1 cup	36
Tamales (Wolf)	scant cup	68
Taquitos, Beef, Shredded, with Guacamole, frozen (Van de Kamp's)	8 oz	100
Tostada, Beef, Supreme, frozen (Van de Kamp's)	8½ oz	350
Tuna Helper, Country Dumplings, Noodles 'n Tuna (Betty Crocker), with added ingredients	⅕ pkg	40
Tuna Helper, Creamy Noodles 'n Tuna (Betty Crocker), with added ingredients	⅕ pkg	20
Tuna Helper, Noodles, Cheese Sauce 'n Tuna (Betty Crocker), with added ingredients	⅕ pkg	40

**Contains less than 20 milligrams of calcium.*

Food	*Portion*	*Calcium (mg)*
Prepared Main Dishes, *continued*		
Tuna Helper, Tuna Tetrazzini (Betty Crocker), with added ingredients	1/5 pkg	60
Tuna Noodle Casserole (Stouffer's)	5 3/4 oz	80
Tuna salad with celery, salad dressing (mayo-type), pickle, onion, and egg	1 cup	41
Turkey (Banquet)	1 dinner	98
Turkey, Breast of, Sliced, with Mushrooms, frozen dinner, Le Menu (Swanson)	1 dinner	40
Turkey Casserole with Gravy and Dressing (Stouffer's)	9 3/4 oz	100
Turkey, Chunky, frozen pie (Swanson)	1 pie	20
Turkey, Extra Helping Dinner (Banquet)	19 oz	176
Turkey, frozen dinner, Hungry-Man (Swanson)	1 dinner	80
Turkey, frozen dinner (Swanson)	1 dinner	40
Turkey, frozen entree, Hungry-Man (Swanson)	1 entree	40
Turkey, frozen entree (Swanson)	1 entree	20
Turkey, frozen meat pie, Hungry-Man (Swanson)	1 pie	40
Turkey, frozen meat pie (Swanson)	1 pie	20
Turkey Pie (Stouffer's)	10 oz	80

Food	Portion	Calcium (mg)
Prepared Main Dishes, *continued*		
Turkey Tetrazzini (Stouffer's)	6 oz	60
Turkey with Gravy, frozen main course entree (Swanson)	1 entree	20
Veal Parmigiana, Dinner Classics (Armour)	1 dinner	100
Veal Parmigiana, Extra Helping Dinner (Banquet)	20 oz	249
Veal Parmigiana, Family Entree (Banquet)	6.4 oz	92
Veal Parmigiana, frozen dinner, Hungry-Man (Swanson)	1 dinner	200
Veal Parmigiana, frozen dinner (Swanson)	1 dinner	150
Veal Parmigiana, International Favorites Cookin' Bag Entrees (Banquet)	5 oz	144
Veal Parmigiana, International Favorites Dinners (Banquet)	11 oz	121
Veal Patties, Breaded, Entree Express (Banquet)	3 oz	23
Welsh Rarebit (Stouffer's)	5 oz	400
Western American Favorites Dinners (Banquet)	1 dinner	93
Western-Style frozen dinner, Hungry-Man (Swanson)	1 dinner	80
Western-Style frozen dinner (Swanson)	1 dinner	60

Food	Portion	Calcium (mg)
Candies, *continued*		
M&M's Peanut Chocolate Candies	1.67 oz	40
M&M's Plain Chocolate Candies	1.69 oz	80
Mars Bar	1.76 oz	80
Milk Chocolate Bar (Hershey's)	1.45 oz	80
Milk Chocolate Bar, with Almonds (Hershey's)	1.45 oz	80
Milky Way Bar (M&M/Mars)	2.1 oz	60
Mint Parfait (Pearson's)	1 oz	20
Mister Goodbar Chocolate Bar (Hershey's)	1.65 oz	40
Mounds Bar (Peter Paul)	1.65	*
Munch Peanut Bar (M&M/Mars)	1.42 oz	20
Peanut Butter Parfait (Pearson's)	1 oz	20
Peanuts, Chocolate Covered (Nabisco)	1 oz	20
Peppermint Pattie (York)	1.25 oz	*
Powerhouse (Peter Paul)	2 oz	40
Raisins, Chocolate Covered (Nabisco)	1 oz	20
Reese's Peanut Butter Cups (Hershey's)	1.60 oz	20
Reese's Pieces (Hershey's)	1.75 oz	40
Sesame seed candies—See Halvah Candies		
Snickers Bar (M&M/Mars)	2 oz	60
Stars, Chocolate, Milk (Nabisco)	1 oz	40

**Contains less than 20 milligrams of calcium.*

Food	*Portion*	*Calcium (mg)*
Candies, *continued*		
Twix Caramel Cookie Bars (M&M/Mars)	2.06 oz.	20
Twix Peanut Butter Cookie Bars (M&M/Mars)	1.89 oz	20
Wispa (Peter Paul)	1 oz	60
SNACKS		
Bars, Breakfast, Chocolate Chip (Carnation)	1.44 oz	20
Bars, Breakfast, Chocolate Crunch (Carnation)	1.34 oz	20
Bars, Breakfast, Honey Nut (Carnation)	1.35 oz	20
Bars, Breakfast, Peanut Butter Crunch (Carnation)	1.35 oz	20
Bars, Breakfast, Peanut Butter with Chocolate Chips (Carnation)	1.39 oz	20
Bars, Chocolate Chip (Slender/Carnation)	2 bars	250
Bars, Chocolate Peanut Butter (Slender/Carnation)	2 bars	250
Bars, Chocolate (Slender/Carnation)	2 bars	250
Bars, Milk Break, Chocolate (Pillsbury)	1 bar	150
Bars, Milk Break, Natural Flavor (Pillsbury)	1 bar	150
Bars, Milk Break, Peanut Butter (Pillsbury)	1 bar	150
Chips, Corn, Planters (Nabisco)	1 oz	40
Chips, Corn (Flavor Tree)	1 oz	40

Food	Portion	Calcium (mg)
Snacks, *continued*		
Chips, Tortilla, Nacho Flavor, Planters (Nabisco)	1 oz	40
Chips, Tortilla, Traditional, Planters, (Nabisco)	1 oz	40
Crackers, Cheese and Peanut Butter Sandwich (Nabisco)	1/2 oz	20
Crackers, Cheese Ritz (Nabisco)	1/2 oz	20
Crackers, Cheese 'n Chive Snack, Dip in a Chip	1/2 oz	20
Crackers, Low Salt, Ritz (Nabisco)	1/2 oz	20
Crackers, Milk, Royal Lunch (Nabisco)	1/2 oz	20
Crackers, Ritz (Nabisco)	1/2 oz	20
Crackers, Round Toast, Planters (Nabisco)	1 oz	20
Crackers, Saltine, Premium (Nabisco)	1/2 oz	20
Crackers, Sesame and Cheese Snack Sticks, Twigs (Nabisco)	1/2 oz	40
Crackers, Sesame Baked Crispy Snacks, Great Crisps! (Nabisco)	1/2 oz	20
Crackers, Sesame Bread Wafers, Meal Mates (Nabisco)	1/2 oz	20
Crackers, Snack Vegetable Thins (Nabisco)	1/2 oz	40
Crackers, Sociables (Nabisco)	1/2 oz	20

Food	Portion	Calcium (mg)
Snacks, *continued*		
Granola Bars, Chocolate Chip Granola Dipps (Quaker)	1 bar	29
Granola Bar, Cinnamon (Nature Valley)	1 bar	20
Granola Bar, Cocoa Creme, Chocolate Covered, New Trail (Hershey's)	1.3 oz	40
Granola Bar, Coconut (Nature Valley)	1 bar	20
Granola Bar, Honey Graham, Chocolate Covered, New Trail (Hershey's)	1.3 oz	20
Granola Bar, Peanut Butter Flavor, Chocolate Covered, New Trail (Hershey's)	1.3 oz	40
Granola Bar, Peanut Butter/Chocolate Chip, New Trail (Hershey's)	1.4 oz	20
Granola Bars, Rocky Road Granola Dipps (Quaker)	1 bar	30
Granola Clusters, Almond (Nature Valley)	1 roll	20
Granola Clusters, Apple Cinnamon (Nature Valley)	1 roll	20
Granola Clusters, Caramel (Nature Valley)	1 roll	40
Granola Clusters, Chocolate Chip (Nature Valley)	1 roll	20

Food	Portion	Calcium (mg)
Snacks, *continued*		
Granola Clusters, Chocolate (Nature Valley)	1 roll	40
Melba Toast, Sesame Rounds (Old London)	5 rounds	20
Party Mix (Flavor Tree)	1 oz	60
Party Mix, No Salt Added (Flavor Tree)	1 oz	40
Peanut Butter Sandwich, Toasted (Nabisco)	1/2 oz	20
Potato Chips, Regular (Pringles)	1 oz	*
Potato Chips, Rippled (Pringles)	1 oz	*
Potato Chips, Sour Cream 'N Onion (Pringles)	1 oz	*
Sesame Chips (Flavor Tree)	1 oz	60
Sesame Crunch (Flavor Tree)	1 oz	*
Sesame Sticks (Flavor Tree)	1 oz	60
Sesame Sticks, No Salt Added (Flavor Tree)	1 oz	60
Sesame Sticks, with bran (Flavor Tree)	1 oz	60
Snack Sticks, Cheese (Pepperidge Farm)	8 crackers	20
Snacks, Cheese Flavored, Cheese 'N Crunch (Nabisco)	1 oz	20
Snacks, Cheese, Zesty Doo Dads (Nabisco)	1 oz	20
Snacks, Original Doo Dads (Nabisco)	1 oz	20

**Contains less than 20 milligrams of calcium.*

Food	*Portion*	*Calcium (mg)*
NUTS		
Almonds, blanched, natural, sliced (Planters)	1 oz	60
Almonds, dried, blanched	1 oz	70
Almonds, dry-roasted	1 oz	80
Almonds, dry-roasted (Planters)	1 oz	80
Almonds, oil-roasted	1 oz	66
Almonds, oil-roasted, blanched	1 oz	55
Almonds, smoked (Planters)	1 oz	60
Almonds, toasted, unblanched	1 oz	80
Brazil Nuts, dried, unblanched	1 oz	50
Cashew Nuts, dry-roasted, wholes and halves	1 cup	62
Cashew Nuts, oil-roasted, wholes and halves	1 cup	53
Filberts or Hazelnuts, dried, blanched	1 oz	55
Filberts or Hazelnuts, dried, unblanched	1 oz	53
Filberts or Hazelnuts, dry-roasted, unblanched	1 oz	55
Filberts or Hazelnuts, oil-roasted, unblanched	1 oz	56
Macadamia Nuts, dried	1 oz	20
Macadamia Nuts, oil-roasted, wholes or halves	1 cup	60
Mixed Nuts, Deluxe, oil-roasted (Planters)	1 oz	20
Mixed nuts, dry-roasted (Planters)	1 oz	20

Food	*Portion*	*Calcium (mg)*
Nuts, *continued*		
Mixed Nuts, oil-roasted (Planters)	1 oz	20
Peanut butter, chunky (Jif)	2 tbsp	*
Peanut butter, creamy (Jif)	2 tbsp	*
Peanut Butter, crunchy (Bama)	2 tbsp	20
Peanuts, roasted in shell, salted (Planters)	1 oz	20
Peanuts, roasted in shell, unsalted (Planters)	1 oz	20
Peanuts, Sweet 'N Crunchy (Planters)	1 oz	20
Pecans, chips, halves, pieces (Planters)	1 oz	20
Pecans, dried, halves	1 cup	39
Pecans, dry-roasted	2 oz	20
Pecans, oil-roasted	1 cup	37
Pistachio Nuts, dried	1 oz	38
Pistachio Nuts, dry-roasted	1 oz	20
Pistachios, dry-roasted (Planters)	1 oz	20
Pistachios, Red (Planters)	1 oz	20
Pistachios, salted (Planters)	1 oz	20
Sesame Nut Mix, oil-roasted (Planters)	1 oz	20
Sunflower Nuts, dry-roasted (Planters)	1 oz	20
Sunflower Nuts, oil-roasted (Planters)	1 oz	20
Sunflower Nuts, unsalted, dry-roasted (Planters)	1 oz	20
Sunflower Seeds (Planters)	1 oz	20
Walnuts, Black (Planters)	1 oz	20
Walnuts, English	1 oz	27

**Contains less than 20 milligrams of calcium.*

BEVERAGES AND JUICES

Food	*Portion*	*Calcium (mg)*
Apple Juice	1 cup	16
Beer	12 oz.	18
Breakfast, Instant, Chocolate (Carnation)	1.26 oz	100
Breakfast, Instant, Chocolate Mix (Pillsbury) with 8 oz milk	1 pouch	250
Breakfast, Instant, Chocolate Malt (Carnation)	1.21 oz	100
Breakfast, Instant, Chocolate Malt Mix (Pillsbury) with 8 oz milk	1 pouch	250
Breakfast, Instant, Coffee (Carnation)	1.26 oz	100
Breakfast, Instant, Eggnog (Carnation)	1.21 oz	100
Breakfast, Instant, Strawberry (Carnation)	1.25 oz	100
Breakfast, Instant, Vanilla (Carnation)	1.24 oz	100
Carrot Juice, canned	½ cup	29
Chocolate Milk—See Milk		

Food	*Portion*	*Calcium (mg)*
Cocoa, Hot Chocolate, and Mini-Marshmallows instant mix packets (Carnation)	1 oz	54
Cocoa, Hot Chocolate, Milk, instant mix packets (Carnation)	1 oz	89
Cocoa, Hot Chocolate, Milk, Mix, reconstituted (Swiss Miss)	6 oz	40
Cocoa, Hot Chocolate, Rich, 70 calorie mix packets (Carnation)	1 envelope	89
Cocoa, Hot Chocolate, Rich, instant mix packets (Carnation)	1 oz	55
Cocoa, Hot, Double Rich Mix, reconstituted (Swiss Miss)	6 oz	40
Cocoa, Hot, Lite Mix, reconstituted (Swiss Miss)	6 oz	60
Cocoa, Hot, Sugar Free Mix (Swiss Miss)	15 grams	120
Cocoa, Hot, Sugar Free Mix (Carnation)	1 envelope or 4 heaping tsp	123
Cocoa, Hot, with Marshmallow Flavor, Sugar Free Mix (Swiss Miss)	15 grams	120
Coffee, ground (Folger's)	1 tbsp grounds	7
Coffee, instant, decaffeinated (High Point)	1 tsp powder	3
Coffee, instant (Folger's)	1 tsp powder	3
Coffee Whitener, nondairy, liquid	½ cup	11

Food	*Portion*	*Calcium (mg)*
Coffee Whitener, nondairy, powdered	1 cup	21
Cranberry Juice Cocktail, bottled	1 cup	8
Grape Juice	1 cup	22
Grapefruit Juice	1 cup	22
Juice drinks, aseptic (Sunkist), all flavors	8.45 fl oz	*
Milk—See Dairy and Egg Products		
Orange Juice, canned	1 cup	21
Orange Juice (Sunkist)	6 fl oz	*
Orange Juice (Citrus Hill)	6 fl oz	*
Orange Juice, frozen, concentrate, diluted	1 cup	22
Orange Juice, frozen, concentrate (Sunkist)	6 fl oz	*
Pineapple Juice, canned	1 cup	42
Pineapple Juice, frozen, concentrate, diluted	1 cup	28
Pineapple Juice, unsweetened (Del Monte)	6 fl oz	20
Prune Juice, canned	1 cup	30
Sauerkraut Juice, canned	1 cup	80
Tomato and Chile Cocktail (Del Monte)	6 fl oz	20
Tomato Juice (Campbell's)	6 oz	*
Tomato Juice, canned	6 fl oz	16
Tomato Juice (Hunt's)	6 oz	20
Vegetable Juice V-8	6 oz	20
Vegetable Juice V-8, No-Salt-Added	6 oz	20
Vegetable Juice V-8, Spicy Hot	6 oz	20
Wine, Table	3 ½ fl oz	9

**Contains less than 20 milligrams of calcium.*

FAST FOOD AND PIZZA

Food	*Portion*	*Calcium (mg)*
ARBY'S		
Bac 'n Cheddar Deluxe Sandwich	1 each	100
Baked Potato, Plain	1 each (11 oz)	20
Beef 'n Cheddar Sandwich	1 each	80
Chicken Breast Sandwich	1 each	100
Ham 'n Cheese, Hot, Sandwich	1 each	200
Junior Roast Beef Sandwich	1 each	40
King Roast Beef Sandwich	1 each	100
Regular Roast Beef Sandwich	1 each	80
Shake, Chocolate	1 each	300
Shake, Jamocha	1 each	300
Shake, Vanilla	1 each	300
Super Roast Beef Sandwich	1 each	100
Superstuffed Potato, Broccoli and Cheddar	1 each	150
Superstuffed Potato, Deluxe	1 each	300
Superstuffed Potato, Mushroom and Cheese	1 each	300
Superstuffed Potato, Taco	1 each	450
Turkey Deluxe Sandwich	1 each	80

Food	Portion	Calcium (mg)
ARTHUR TREACHER'S		
Chicken Sandwich	1 each	59
Chowder	6 oz	61
Coleslaw	1 order	24
Fish Sandwich	1 each	89
Shrimp	7 pieces	57
BURGER CHEF		
Big Shef	1 each	178
Cheeseburger	1 each	145
Cheeseburger, Double	1 each	218
Chicken Club	1 each	77
Fisherman's Filet	1 each	146
Fun Meal	1 each	84
Hamburger	1 each	75
Mushroom Burger	1 each	262
Super Shef	1 each	241
TOP Shef	1 each	226
BURGER KING		
Cheeseburger	1 each	150
Cheeseburger, Double	1 each	250
Cheeseburger, Double, Bacon	1 each	226
Chicken Sandwich Specialty	1 each	60
Ham and Cheese Sandwich Specialty	1 each	250
Hamburger	1 each	60
Hamburger, Double	1 each	60
Milk, Homogenized	1 each	300
Shake, Chocolate	1 each	250
Shake, Vanilla	1 each	300
Veal Parmigiana Sandwich	1 each	300
Whaler Sandwich	1 each	80
Whaler Sandwich with Cheese	1 each	200
Whopper Jr. Sandwich	1 each	60

Food	Portion	Calcium (mg)
Burger King, *Continued*		
Whopper Jr. Sandwich with Cheese	1 each	150
Whopper Sandwich	1 each	100
Whopper Sandwich, Double Beef	1 each	100
Whopper Sandwich, Double Beef, with Cheese	1 each	300
Whopper Sandwich with Cheese	1 each	250
DOMINO'S		
Cheese Pizza, 12-inch	2 slices	300
Cheese Pizza, 16-inch	2 slices	400
Pepperoni Pizza, 12-inch	2 slices	300
Pepperoni Pizza, 16-inch	2 slices	400
HARDEE'S		
Apple Turnover	1 serving	19
Big Deluxe	1 sandwich	98
Big Roast Beef	1 serving	74
Biscuit	1 serving	149
Biscuit, Bacon and Egg	1 serving	144
Biscuit, Cinnamon 'N' Raisin	1 serving	89
Biscuit Gravy	1 serving	168
Biscuit, Ham	1 serving	181
Biscuit, Ham and Egg	1 serving	211
Biscuit, Sausage	1 serving	134
Biscuit, Sausage and Egg	1 serving	169
Biscuit, Steak	1 serving	121
Biscuit, Steak and Egg	1 serving	151
Biscuit with Egg	1 serving	179
Biscuit with jelly	1 serving	153
Cheeseburger	1 sandwich	123
Cheeseburger, Bacon	1 sandwich	152
Chicken Fillet	1 serving	83
Egg, Fried, medium, one	1 serving	30

Food	Portion	Calcium (mg)
Hardee's, *Continued*		
Fisherman's Fillet	1 serving	139
French Fries, Large	1 serving	21
Hamburger	1 sandwich	23
Hot Dog	1 sandwich	43
Ham 'N' Cheese, Hot	1 serving	207
Milk, Whole	½ pint	298
Milk Shake	1 serving	450
Mushroom 'N' Swiss	1 serving	111
Roast Beef Sandwich	1 sandwich	56
Salad, Chef	1 serving	212
Salad, Shrimp	1 serving	104
Turkey Club	1 serving	39
JACK IN THE BOX		
Breakfast Jack	1 serving	170
Burger, Swiss and Bacon	1 sandwich	230
Cheeseburger	1 sandwich	160
Cheeseburger, Bacon, Supreme	1 sandwich	310
Chicken Strips Dinner	1 serving	110
Chicken Supreme	1 serving	240
Crescent Sausage	1 serving	170
Crescent Supreme	1 serving	150
Eggs, Scrambled, Breakfast	1 serving	250
Ham 'N Cheese, Hot	1 serving	310
Hamburger	1 sandwich	70
Jumbo Jack	1 sandwich	100
Jumbo Jack with Cheese	1 sandwich	250
Milk	1 serving	250
Moby Jack	1 serving	160
Nachos, Cheese	1 serving	370
Nachos Supreme	1 serving	410
Onion Rings	1 serving	30
Orange Juice	1 serving	20
Pancake Breakfast	1 serving	100

Food	Portion	Calcium (mg)
Jack in the Box, *Continued*		
Pita, Club	1 serving	80
Shake, Chocolate	1 serving	350
Shake, Strawberry	1 serving	350
Shake, Vanilla	1 serving	350
Shrimp Dinner	1 serving	370
Shrimp Salad	1 serving	100
Sirloin Steak Dinner	1 serving	220
Taco, Regular	1 serving	100
Taco Salad	1 serving	280
McDONALD'S		
Big Mac	1 sandwich	203
Biscuit, plain	1 serving	74
Biscuit with Sausage	1 serving	82
Biscuit with Sausage and Egg	1 serving	119
Cheeseburger	1 sandwich	169
Cones	1 serving	183
Cookies, Chocolaty Chip	1 box	29
Egg McMuffin	1 sandwich	226
Eggs, Scrambled	1 serving	61
Filet-O-Fish	1 sandwich	133
Hamburger	1 sandwich	84
Hotcakes with butter, syrup	1 serving	103
McD.L.T.	1 sandwich	230
Milk Shake, Chocolate	1 serving	320
Milk Shake, Strawberry	1 serving	322
Milk Shake, Vanilla	1 serving	329
Muffin, English, with butter	1 serving	117
Quarter Pounder	1 sandwich	98
Quarter Pounder with Cheese	1 sandwich	255
Sausage	1 serving	16
Sausage McMuffin	1 serving	168

Food	*Portion*	*Calcium (mg)*
McDonald's, *Continued*		
Sausage McMuffin with Egg	1 serving	196
Sundae, Caramel (Carmel)	1 serving	200
Sundae, Fudge, Hot	1 serving	215
Sundae, Strawberry	1 serving	174
ROY ROGERS		
Bacon Cheeseburger	1 each	343
Bar Burger	1 each	343
Cheeseburger	1 each	340
Chicken Breast	1 each	35
Chicken Breast & Wing	1 each	52
Chicken Thigh & Leg	1 each	27
Coleslaw	1 order	34
Crescent Roll	1 each	52
Roast Beef Sandwich	1 each	87
Roast Beef Sandwich, Large	1 each	89
Roast Beef Sandwich, Large, with Cheese	1 each	339
Roast Beef Sandwich with Cheese	1 each	337
Shake, Chocolate	1 each	290
Shake, Strawberry	1 each	284
Shake, Vanilla	1 each	300
Strawberry Shortcake	1 each	274
WENDY'S		
American Cheese	1 slice	100
Breakfast Sandwich	1 each	150
Cheeseburger (Single Hamburger with American Cheese), on multi-grain wheat bun	1 each	120

Food	Portion	Calcium (mg)
Wendy's, *Continued*		
Cheeseburger (Single Hamburger with American Cheese), on white bun	1 each	140
Cheeseburger with Bacon on white bun	1 each	150
Chicken Sandwich on multi-grain wheat bun	1 each	20
Chili	8 oz	80
Danish	1 piece	20
French Toast	2 slices	80
Frosty Dairy Dessert	12 fl oz	300
Hamburger, Double, on white bun	1 each	40
Hamburger, Kids' Meal	1 each	20
Hamburger, Single, on multi-grain wheat bun	1 each	20
Hamburger, Single, on white bun	1 each	40
Home Fries	1 order	20
Hot Chocolate	6 fl oz	20
Hot Stuffed Baked Potato, Bacon & Cheese	1 each	200
Hot Stuffed Baked Potato, Broccoli & Cheese	1 each	250
Hot Stuffed Baked Potato, Cheese	1 each	350
Hot Stuffed Baked Potato, Chicken a la King	1 each	60
Hot Stuffed Baked Potato, Chili & Cheese	1 each	250
Hot Stuffed Baked Potato, Plain	1 each (8.8 oz)	20
Hot Stuffed Baked Potato, Sour Cream & Chives	1 each	40

Food	Portion	Calcium (mg)
Wendy's, *Continued*		
Hot Stuffed Baked Potato, Stroganoff & Sour Cream	1 each	80
Milk	8 fl oz	300
Milk,Chocolate	8 fl oz	300
Omelet, Ham & Cheese	1 each	100
Omelet, Ham, Cheese, & Mushroom	1 each	100
Omelet, Ham, Cheese, Onion, Green Pepper	1 each	150
Omelet, Mushroom, Onion, Green Pepper	1 each	60
Salad Bar, Garden Spot, American Cheese, Imitation	1 oz	200
Salad Bar, Garden Spot, Broccoli	½ cup	20
Salad Bar, Garden Spot, Cheddar Cheese, Imitation	1 oz	200
Salad Bar, Garden Spot, Coleslaw	½ cup	20
Salad Bar, Garden Spot, Cottage Cheese	½ cup	60
Salad Bar, Garden Spot, Pasta Salad	½ cup	20
Salad Bar, Garden Spot, Sunflower Seeds & Raisins	1 cup	40
Salad, Side, Pick-Up Window	1 each	100
Salad, Taco	1 each	200
Scrambled Eggs	1 order	60
Toast with margarine	2 slices	20